CORE
PERFORMANCE

**THE REVOLUTIONARY WORKOUT PROGRAM
TO TRANSFORM YOUR BODY AND YOUR LIFE**

MARK VERSTEGEN
AND PETE WILLIAMS

FOREWORD BY
NOMAR GARCIAPARRA

RODALE

© 2004 by Joxy LLC

First published 2004
First published in paperback 2005

All rights reserved. No part of this publication may be reproduced or transmitted in any form or by any means, electronic or mechanical, including photocopying, recording, or any other information storage and retrieval system, without the written permission of the publisher.

Printed in the United States of America
Rodale Inc. makes every effort to use acid-free ⊗, recycled paper ♻.

Photo credit information appears on page 276.

Book design by Joanna Williams

Library of Congress Cataloging-in-Publication Data

Verstegen, Mark, date.
  Core performance : the revolutionary workout program to transform your body and your life / by Mark Verstegen and Pete Williams ; foreword by Nomar Garciaparra.
     p.   cm.
  Includes index.
  ISBN-13 978–1–57954–908–4 hardcover
  ISBN-10 1–57954–908–X hardcover
  ISBN-13 978–1–59486–168–0 paperback
  ISBN-10 1–59486–168–4 paperback
  1. Bodybuilding. 2. Exercise. I. Williams, Pete, date. II. Title.
GV546.5.V47   2004
613.7'1—dc22   2003022833

Distributed to the trade by Holtzbrinck Publishers

    6 8 10 9 7 5   hardcover
       8 10 9 7   paperback

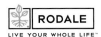

For Amy
—M.V.

For Suzy and Luke
—P.W.

CONTENTS

PART 4: THE CORE LIFE PLAN

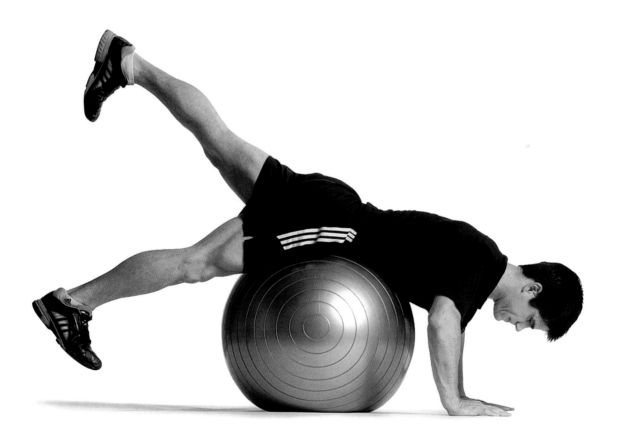

WWW.COREPERFORMANCE.COM

ACKNOWLEDGMENTS

This book is part of an ongoing process of learning to evolve continually in all aspects of life. I want to thank everyone who has helped me develop the knowledge, programs, and passion reflected in these pages. To list everyone by name would have required at least half the space we have in this book, but I wanted to single out the following:

- To Mom and Dad, for providing the love and nurturing that's been the pillar strength of my life. I hope I'm a living example of all that you represent and all that you've taught me. To my extended family, both related and not, for being such inspirational role models and molding me into the person I am now and will be in the future.

- To my late mentor Coach K. and Sara Kruckenberg, both of whom finished sharing the meaning of life with me far sooner than I would have liked. I am driven each day by your example. Friends, indeed, are the flowers in the garden of life.

- To those who train at Athletes' Performance, every one of you is a continual source of inspiration and deserving of our endless pursuit of excellence. To the staff and extended community of Athletes' Performance, I hope I motivate and inspire you to the degree you have done so for me. It is an incredible honor to represent all of you.

- To fellow collaborators David Black, Pete Williams, and Craig Friedman, thanks for sharing my vision. To Lou Schuler, Jeremy Katz, and the entire team at Rodale, thanks for helping me bring my message to others.

- And to my wife, Amy, for all of your endless support and for exceeding my wildest expectations of what love, joy, and friendship two people can share. I'm blessed each day. You are my core.

FOREWORD

BY NOMAR GARCIAPARRA

For the last 10 years, I've followed *Core Performance*. This program, along with Mark Verstegen's guidance and motivational skills, has transformed me from a skinny, 155-pound college baseball player with little power into one of the best-conditioned players in Major League Baseball.

Each January, I report to Mark's Athletes' Performance training center in Arizona for 6 weeks of intense training. During this time, I perform a lengthier, more intense version of the Core Workout in order to get ready for a grueling baseball season.

The rest of the year, I follow a program very similar to the one you'll find on the coming pages. It takes me 45 minutes to an hour each day, requires minimal equipment, and gives me a better total-body workout than any other program available. Even though I travel constantly, I find I can do my workout in almost any gym.

The best part of this program is that it's accessible to everyone, not just professional athletes but also kids, working adults, and se-niors. It's designed for men and women. In fact, women seem to get the hang of this program more quickly than men do since women tend to have more natural flexibility, balance, and stability in their bodies.

Mark has recognized that the goal of training is not to look good—although this will transform your body—but rather to condition yourself for powerful, *functional* movement. This includes everything from daily actions like stepping out of a car or lifting a toddler to sport-specific moves like swinging a golf club or a tennis racket.

Most workout programs are based on bodybuilding and designed solely to help you look better. The focus is on losing weight, developing muscle, and looking good at the beach. There's nothing wrong with that, of course. In fact, if you follow this program, you're going to be in the best shape of your life. The difference is that you're going to be quicker, stronger, and fitter; have greater flexibility; and be able to generate more power throughout your body. You'll have functional strength that can be put to use.

With most workout programs, you train individual body parts with the goal of producing larger muscles. But the problem is you don't become any more flexible. You might gain strength, but you don't build power, the ability to generate force behind your movements. You spend a ton of time building showy muscles, such as the biceps and triceps, while ignoring all of the vital little muscles that support your hips, torso, shoulders, and back.

These areas make up pillar strength, the basis of all movement. We tend to "lose" these muscles if we don't use them, which is why so many people end up with devastating hip, back, and rotator cuff problems. Mark is fond of referring to pillar strength as your body's suspension system. Without it, your body will not withstand the demands of daily life and will rapidly deteriorate as you age.

But if you can build that strong suspension system, you can avoid many of those long-term problems while improving the quality of your life right now.

I've seen successful business executives work with Mark and develop better flexibility and torque in their golf swings. People find that they can leap higher in pickup basketball games and improve their endurance and lateral movement for tennis. Others discover that they can have greater flexibility and power for karate. Former high school athletes, now in their thirties, forties, or fifties, realize they not only can combat the effects of aging but also can improve their performances.

Older folks have worked with Mark to regain movement they thought was gone forever. Kids establish positive workout habits, which is important at a time when children are exercising less and less. Everyone benefits from increased energy and the mental power that comes from constantly improving.

Even if you're active and work out, I bet you're still ignoring these core areas. I know this because I often go into gyms where these huge guys are lifting 100-pound dumbbells. I'll grab a 5-pound weight, and they'll kind of chuckle and wonder what possible benefit I could derive from it. I'll explain that I'm working these little muscles in my shoulders that I use in my sport and in daily life. I might show them another lift with a little dumbbell that they can't do because it requires a degree of flexibility or balance they don't have. Maybe I'm using a muscle group they've been ignoring. Or I might be doing a pushup or a situp by using a big rubber physioball that requires a degree of balance.

Maybe you're the type of person who hates working out. You find it boring, tedious, and even a little embarrassing to be around people who look more fit and powerful. Believe me, I know how you feel. As a gangly college baseball player at Georgia Tech, I hated working out. I figured I could hit the ball and field well. Why did I have to worry about conditioning?

I would see these massive football players lifting heavy weights and feel embarrassed. I couldn't even bench-press a 45-pound bar with no weights on it. Mark was working at Georgia Tech at the time, and he sensed my frustration. He pulled me aside one day and had me perform a few exercises that emphasized flexibility and balance over brute strength.

When I was done, he nodded toward the football players. "Those guys can't do what you just did."

Mark showed me how to develop my core stability, my body's suspension system. Everything we did was to make me more flexible, balanced, and more powerful. Notice I said *more powerful*, not stronger. I became stronger, of course, but the focus was on creating as much power and force as possible. Bodybuilders tend to be very big, but they have little power. They can lift heavy weights, but they can't generate a lot of force with a tennis racket or a golf club because they don't work all of those little muscles. They have little flexibility.

Over the years, I've increased my weight from 155 to 190. I'm lean and you'd probably call me ripped, but I'm not muscle-bound or bulky. In fact, I don't look like someone who weighs 190. A pound of fat takes up more space than a pound of lean muscle, which is why I can stand next to a guy who's my same height and weight and look smaller. But pound for pound, I can generate as much force as anyone can.

You're not going to gain 35 pounds on this program—unless that's your goal. Mark tweaked the Core Workout for me because I needed the extra bulk to get through the rigors of a 162-game baseball season.

I sometimes find it challenging to match Mark's effort. There are days when I feel sluggish, and there's a temptation to slack off, to do one fewer set or get off the exercise bike a few minutes early. Inevitably, he helps me break through the fatigue because of how hard he works himself. I end up doing an extra set or staying on the bike longer than usual. You won't have him with you, but his knowledge and passion as they are conveyed here will drive you.

One of Mark's great strengths is his teaching ability. He's an expert on exercise physiology, sports science, and performance conditioning, but he takes complex concepts and makes them easy to understand. He not only shows you what to do but also explains why you're doing it. We all have a tendency to just do what we're told when it comes to working out. As kids, we do what our coaches and gym teachers tell us, no questions asked.

Mark wants you to understand the science behind every exercise that you do and every meal that you eat. After reading this book, you'll come away with not only a workout program but also a better understanding of how your body works.

You'll find, as I have, that *Core Performance* is more than a workout plan. It gives you a confidence that extends to other aspects of your life. When you look good and feel powerful, you feel better about yourself. Following this program, you'll be prepared for whatever life throws at you.

Because of the success I've had with this program, I'm often asked about Mark. Everyone wants to know what makes his program successful. Inevitably, I'll talk about his knowledge, drive, and ability to motivate. Sometimes I've wished that I could just hand these curious folks a book that outlines the principles and techniques in a way that would make sense to anyone.

Now I can.

—*Nomar Garciaparra,*
professional baseball player

THE CORE MISSION ■

The mission of *Core Performance* is to provide you with the tools to reach your full potential in all aspects of life through an integrated lifestyle program based on cutting-edge training methods and nutritional research.

The goals of *Core Performance* are:

- To increase the quality and duration of your life by boosting performance, productivity, and well-being.
- To reduce the potential for long-term health problems.
- To motivate you toward achieving success in all areas of your life by providing you with easy-to-follow strategies.

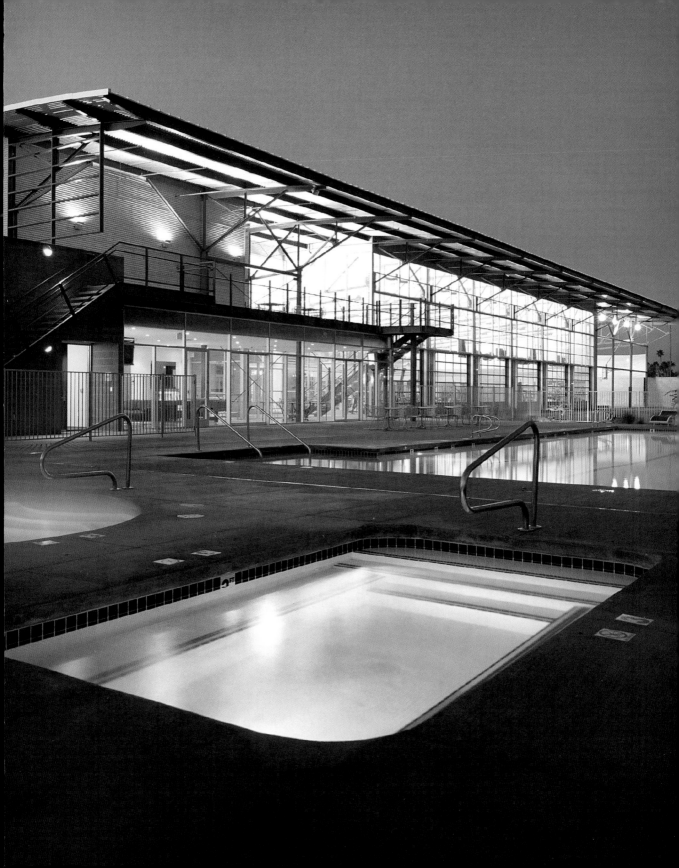

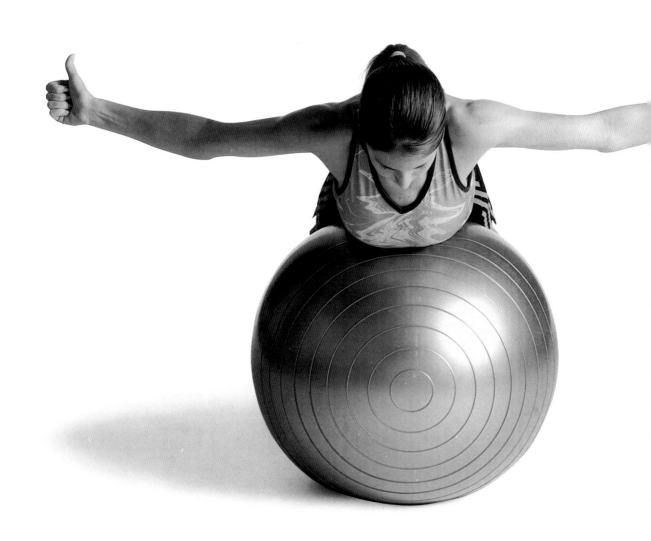

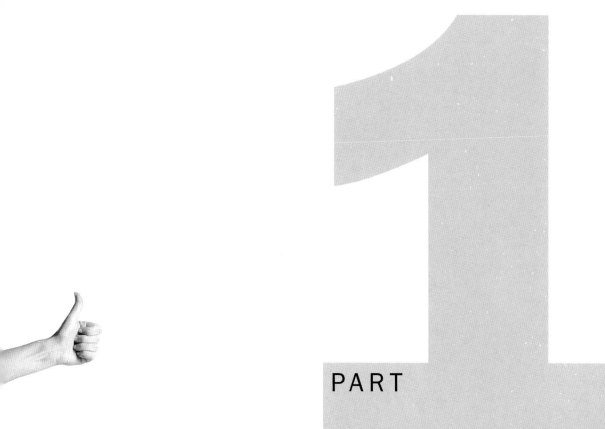

PART

WELCOME TO THE CORE

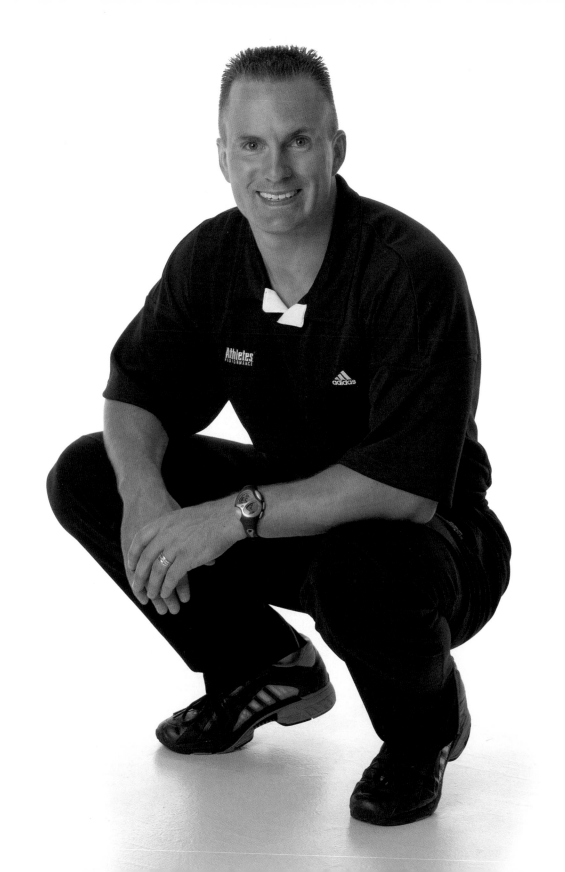

CHAPTER 1

CORE INSPIRATION

Over the past decade, I've helped people from all walks of life perform better—not just in sports but also in their daily lives. I've shown them a program that not only helps them look fitter, it serves as a lifelong formula to maximize performance and help maintain a high quality of life well into their senior years.

You might believe you're already benefiting from a program of diet and exercise. I'm sure you are, to some degree. After all, you've taken the biggest step by committing to better health, and that alone is empowering. But if there's one common denominator I've seen in kids, seniors, working adults—even professional athletes—it's that they do not work out properly, or at least as efficiently as they could. Because of the misinformation they've been fed by the media and marketers, they reap only a fraction of the reward and leave themselves vulnerable to physical ailments down the road.

Take my coauthor, Pete Williams. Pete looks as if he's in decent shape for a guy in his midthirties. He played sports in high school, and now, as a working adult and father, he lifts weights or runs 4 days a week. But he always

has been frustrated by his inability to generate much power, whether it be hitting a baseball or performing martial-arts routines. Despite countless golf lessons, he has found that he cannot get any lift on a ball off the tee.

I asked Pete if he had any physical ailments, and, not surprisingly, he mentioned that his back tightens up while driving. He's constantly squirming in the seat. On long rides, he has to get out and stretch after just an hour.

Not long after he arrived at Athletes' Performance, the cutting-edge training center I own and operate in Tempe, Arizona, I had him hop up on a padded table and lie on his back. I asked him to raise his left leg as high as he could, and he struggled to lift it 45 degrees. I had him put the leg down and then extend it to his left. It barely moved.

I've seen elderly and obese people perform better. By now, some of our interns had gathered around, marveling at this utter lack of flexibility. Professional tennis player Mary Pierce, who happened to be getting stretched and massaged at the next table, casually pulled a leg back so that her toe touched her shoulder.

"There you have it," Pete said, nodding toward Mary. "The difference between a professional athlete and a sportswriter."

"Wrong!" I shouted. I grabbed a rope, wrapped it around Pete's foot, and had him perform the same stretches, this time raising his leg up on his own, then moving it farther by gently assisting with the rope for 2 seconds while exhaling at the end of the stretch. I helped him push at the end, and after just 10 challenging minutes, Pete was able to lift each of his legs nearly 90 degrees.

For 20 years, Pete has been under the impression that he could not physically stretch his hamstrings more than 45 degrees. As a result, his performance in sports suffered, and he developed back problems. But after 10 minutes of our program, he learned that there was no reason he could not—with work—become as flexible as he wanted to be.

The following day, Pete was working out alongside baseball star Roberto Alomar, performing the identical strength and movement routines. Pete still had a long way to go to improve his flexibility, but by seeing what he could

do in such a short time the previous day, he had gained the confidence to do more. In less than 24 hours, Pete had transformed from a sportswriter who interviewed Robbie to an athlete who could train with him. Pete will never play in the major leagues, of course, but there's no reason he can't develop the same flexibility, joint stability, and physical power of an elite athlete.

This program was originally designed to help professional athletes, but anyone can benefit from the same techniques, which you'll learn in this book. Obviously, you don't have the same amount of time to devote to training as a pro athlete, which is why we've streamlined the program. We like to think of this book as our "greatest hits" version. I know my professional athletes will agree with me when I say that if a sportswriter can follow this program, then anyone can.

Pete's like a lot of people who think they're in good shape because they work out regularly and eat right—at least by the standards popularized by fad-diet plans and so-called "experts." In reality, if Pete hadn't made some dramatic changes, he was looking at serious back problems down the road—and there are few physical ailments that hinder you in life like a bad back.

Except maybe hip problems. Pete's hips were so tight and inflexible that he might have one day needed a hip replacement. He might have thrown out his back picking up his infant son. It was obvious why he couldn't drive a baseball, hit a golf ball, or deliver powerful karate kicks; his body was incapable of performing these core movements.

No amount of batting practice or golf lessons can compensate for a body that can't perform functional movements. Poor Pete. Since childhood, he had been lifting weights, running, and knocking himself out on the driving range and in the batting cage, when what he really needed was to work on his *pillar strength,* developing the muscles around the hips, lower back, torso, abs, and shoulder blades.

The worst part of it is that Pete has a tremendous work ethic and probably thought he just had to work harder to perform better. He followed what he thought were sound training methods that, indeed, gave him a degree of muscle, fitness, and endurance. But by training body parts instead of body *movements*—the area we focus on in our program— not only was he not making the most of his time, he was setting himself up for physical problems in the future.

He needed a better program. Which is where *Core Performance* comes in. Yes, we designed this for professional athletes—they represent the bulk of our business, after all—but this same program will benefit you regardless of where you are in life, what sport you play, or even if you don't play sports at all.

Think of your body as a computer. It's a re-markable piece of hardware. It also comes with a lot of powerful software, much of which we'd like to use better if only we knew how. Like a computer, the body comes down with viruses and glitches in its programming that slow it down. *Core Performance* shows you how to best program all of your software to get the most out of the hardware while ridding the body of glitches and viruses so that it operates at maximum power and reaches its ultimate potential.

Everyone I've worked with—from kids and working adults to seniors and pros—has lost body fat, improved flexibility, become more powerful, and strengthened and stabilized his joints. Those who were working out previously found that they were addressing only a fraction of the areas they needed to address in order to maximize performance.

Most important, they discovered that they could make improvements in all of these areas and do it efficiently, in a small block of time, and enjoy the process.

If you're like me, you're not a professional athlete. You're someone with responsibilities, both professional and personal, that create heavy demands on your time. But like an athlete, you have goals, dreams, and a desire to improve. Your body is the vehicle for your success, and I'm here to show you how to make that vehicle run with the most power and efficiency possible.

The main reason I decided to write this

book is that I see a nation of people setting themselves up for long-term problems. We become less active all the time, spending more time in front of the television and the computer. Kids no longer play unless it's an organized activity, and even that's disappearing. Many schools have eliminated physical-education classes.

Working adults have less time to exercise than ever before. As a result, we're seeing an increase in type 2 diabetes, obesity, heart disease, and hip-replacement surgeries. Modern medicine has enabled people to live longer than ever before, but their quality of life is decreasing all the time.

A recent study published in the *Annals of Internal Medicine* revealed that people who are overweight at age 40 are likely to die at least 3 years sooner than those who are not overweight. Other studies suggest that overweight children are likely to be overweight adults. If we don't stop this epidemic, it's possible that life expectancies actually could decrease in the coming years—even with modern medical advances.

When people do commit to a program of nutrition and exercise, it's usually a quick-fix solution that takes pounds off quickly but fails to address these long-term issues. You might end up with a thinner physique (however temporarily), but you'll almost certainly fail to create a body that's more powerful and resistant to injury.

We need to turn our focus away from just looking better. Wouldn't you also like to perform better in all areas of your life?

It's a simple question, I know, but I'm often surprised at the confused looks I get when I talk to people who are considering training with me. They figure I'm going to help them develop a leaner physique and become stronger.

I do that, of course, and that will happen if you commit to this program. But why put in all that time and effort solely to look better and, perhaps, feel better? Wouldn't you rather *perform* better?

Wouldn't you rather experience more success and fulfillment at work? At play? In dealing with your friends and family? Wouldn't you rather have a body that not only looks good but also is capable of thriving in sports and performing the grueling physical tasks of everyday life?

Wouldn't you rather have a body that will resist injury, a body that will be less likely to develop the types of hip and back problems that plague millions of people? Wouldn't you rather follow a nutrition program that will prevent type 2 diabetes and obesity?

Wouldn't you rather have a fit body that's not an end goal but a means to help you establish core values and confidence to reach the highest levels of professional and personal success?

People who follow this program tell me that

they're able to perform movements they never thought possible, and you, too, will find that your body will become more flexible, elastic, and explosive than ever before. You'll find you have more stability, which is to say more support around your joints that comes from working the surrounding little muscles that other training programs ignore. You'll also find you enjoy the process and find it easy to integrate into what you're already doing.

We'll accomplish this by training 3 to 6 days a week, for 30 to 60 minutes a day. The program consists of six core routines plus an element of Energy System Development training—what you probably think of as cardio work. Together, they comprise seven units, and you'll do three or four units—or partial units—a day.

We constantly mix up units to challenge your body. Your body needs continual stimulation to avoid falling into a rut. It also needs to recover, which is why 2 to 3 of your 6 days will be lighter in intensity. You'll look forward to these days—referred to as "active rest," "regeneration," or "reload" days—because you're helping your body recover more quickly and avoiding overtraining, which can lead to injury. The program includes a nutritional component based on science, not on quick-fix weight-loss methods.

You will train your entire body on each exercise day, which might be a new concept if you have followed plans that concentrate on certain body parts on designated days. But because we target so many different areas and systems, there's little danger of overtraining your body.

Why will this occur? Because we train movements, not body parts. Many training programs are based on the one-dimensional movements of bodybuilding, exercises designed solely to build a muscle targeted at winning a contest or pleasing a mirror. There's a lot of pushing and pulling, but rarely are the hips, torso, pelvis, and lower back—the key areas of almost all movement—integrated into the training.

Is it any wonder, then, that so many people suffer hip and lower-back problems? It's because they don't train their bodies for these movements. Unless you're training to win a muscle-and-fitness contest, wouldn't you rather spend your time on a program that makes your body more functional, more resistant to injury, *and* better looking?

I've found that many accomplished athletes don't work out properly until I show them the techniques to become more efficient and to maximize their bodies.

Now, if these athletes are exercising incorrectly, my hunch is that you're probably not making the most of your workouts either. But don't worry. The best part about this plan is that you can quickly learn the same techniques that I've taught them and see dramatic results immediately.

Lots of people work out daily but haven't made improvements in years. They stretch and never become more flexible. They lift the same amount of weight week after week. Instead of focusing on their weaknesses, they continue to work on their strengths, because it makes them feel better. I suppose there's some value in that, but wouldn't you rather turn your weaknesses into strengths?

We need to rediscover and reactivate those core movements that we were born with and see in children. If you watch little kids, you'll see them lunge, twist, crawl, pull, and balance naturally. Somewhere along the line, we stop moving this way and subscribe to workout programs that actually discourage these natural movements.

Core Performance is going to show you the same techniques pro athletes use to maximize performance in sports. The same movements children learn naturally can be used by people like you to craft a more functional body that's leaner, stronger, and more explosive. No matter your age, sex, or athletic involvement, you can create a new body and mental toughness that come from meeting physical challenges and that will propel you to new heights in every element of your life.

Don't get me wrong; you will look great. But in the process you'll make the most of your training time by addressing the structural elements, from joint function to flexibility, mobility, strength, and everything that contributes to

your posture. You'll find that you'll literally start to glide through life with a spring in your step instead of plodding along.

I don't mean that just in terms of how you physically walk, but also in the way that people view you and how you perceive your own abilities to accomplish goals, regardless of the challenge.

This is a training regimen. But it's also a way to prepare for the demands of life. You'll be taught a system to perform better, starting with the first chapter. As we go along, you'll learn the secrets of how to improve your fitness level, but more important, your performance level.

INVESTING IN YOURSELF

Your body is the most important investment of your life, and, fortunately, it's something you have control over. If you don't invest in yourself first, the rest of your life's portfolio will suffer. As much as we want to share ourselves with our family, friends, and professional associates, we cannot do so until we take care of ourselves first.

Isn't it amazing that people take better, more proactive care of their cars than their bodies? We spend big money on a car and do everything to protect that investment from Day One. We dutifully change the oil every 3,000 miles. We rush to the shop at the first sign of trouble. We buy extended warranties and insurance, all because we want to protect an investment we know will most likely provide us no value after 8 to 10 years.

And yet we visit the doctor or think about our health only when things go wrong. Cars and all the other material things won't make a difference if we don't have the quality of life we want. The richest man in the world can't buy health. There has to be an investment of time and effort in a plan—not just any plan, but one that will provide the greatest return on investment.

Many training plans, like automobiles, are short-term investments. You'll get your body looking good for a wedding, reunion, or trip to the beach, but you won't take the measures to ensure that your body will function well for a lifetime. What good is it to look good in your twenties, thirties, and forties if you're struggling with joint problems and not able to move efficiently when you're in your sixties, seventies, and eighties?

This program is the one you've needed, even if you didn't realize it. *Core Performance* is a long-term investment in your productivity and wellness. When it comes to your health, you're either going to pay now or pay much more later, and it's a heck of a lot easier and better to make the proper investment now. Once you wait for an injury to occur, you have a potentially chronic problem to deal with, and it's a long road back from there. You could fall into a downward spiral toward disability, poor

health, and a low quality of life. But if you start now, you can minimize the risk of those problems.

I call this proactive concept *prehabilitation,* or *prehab.* You've no doubt heard of rehabilitation or rehab, the painful, often frustrating regimen of exercises to strengthen an area of the body after injury or surgery. Prehab is a series of exercises, which you will learn in this book, geared toward preventing injuries that require rehab.

You can always buy a new car. Once you ruin your body's original equipment, however, you're in trouble. Think of prehab as your own 3,000-mile maintenance, albeit something you'll do even more often to prevent long-term damage.

When I started working in the performance field, I had little idea of the impact my methods would have beyond the sports realm. Then athletes began telling me how the program changed their mindset and gave them a new approach to every aspect of their lives.

If you are someone who hasn't been working out, this is the perfect place to start. You're a blank canvas, and I'm excited because you haven't developed any bad habits. Whatever your starting point, this program will show you the most efficient path.

Start by tossing aside your preconceived limitations. Take off the blinders and envision what you want to achieve for your body. Don't set ceilings and limitations on what you can do. We have accomplished athletes who come to us and still manage to find new heights through our program. So don't tell me you're incapable.

Please don't get discouraged if this program seems a little awkward to you at first. Like anything new, there's a bit of a learning curve, but this is the straightest shot toward achieving your goals. Every athlete I see, even one who earns tens of millions of dollars, feels a little challenged and intimidated at first. But what makes him successful is that he's willing to make a concerted effort. That's all I'm asking of you.

When athletes arrive at our training center, I have them sign a core covenant pledging maximum effort and commitment to improving quality of life. After all, what's more important than that?

Nothing is accomplished without making a commitment—so do that now. The core covenant is waiting for your signature.

THE CORE COVENANT

Dear Friend:

The purpose of this book is to improve performance. My research and development have been aimed at creating programs to assist you in reaching your goals, regardless of your athletic or competitive background. *Core Performance* is designed to provide you with the proper means to achieve your desired results.

I'm very proud of the athletes I train and have very high expectations for them. At the same time, I stress that as an athlete you are ultimately responsible for your own performance. There- fore, while you are engaged in *Core Performance,* I will expect the following:

- Maximum effort
- Honesty
- Excellence
- Consistency
- Enjoyment of the process

Results aren't guaranteed; they're earned. To be sure you get the most out of your *Core Perfor- mance* experience, I ask that you sign this covenant, stating that you're committed to improving performance and are willing to give maximum effort and be honest with yourself so that we may strive for excellence together.

Athlete's Signature: _____

Mark Verstegen's Signature: _____

CHAPTER 2

CORE BEGINNINGS

'm the youngest of five children born to career educators. At one point during my childhood, I noticed that many of my friends received cash awards based on their report-card grades. We had never done that in my family, but I still came home from school one day and asked my mom how much I would get for my grades.

Mom was slicing some cheese and pickles at the time and didn't even look up. "This is your life," she said matter-of-factly. "If you want to fail all of those classes, go ahead. It's your decision, and you'll have to live with that all your life. You can choose to be successful, or you can choose to fail."

With that, she went back to cutting, probably thinking nothing more of the conversation. But that advice has been the driving force in my life. I'm not the first to say that success is a choice or a mindset, but I believe it. I also believe that success requires a plan.

When I joined the football team at Washington State University, I was undersized for a linebacker. So I became a self-taught expert on how an athlete could compensate for modest size by building strength, explosion, flexibility, and power without the use of illegal and unethical methods such as steroids.

Though my college football career ended with a neck injury in my first game, the disappointment reinforced my desire to study every aspect of the body and human performance, and to develop a program to improve them. *Core Performance* is the result of 15 years of research and development with people from all walks of life, including professional athletes.

Core Performance is a physical training program, to be sure, but it is built on a foundation of core values that define us as people. As we overcome these physical challenges, we realize that we can apply these same values to all of life's obstacles.

After earning a master's degree in exercise physiology at the University of Idaho, I began implementing this performance program in the early 1990s at Georgia Tech, where I was the assistant director of player development under Jay Omer, who became one of my mentors. While there, I began working with a young student athlete named Nomar Garciaparra, who since has won two batting titles for the Boston Red Sox.

In 1994, the International Management Group (IMG) recruited me to create the sports science and performance division of the IMG (formerly Bollettieri) Academies in Bradenton, Florida. Our International Performance Institute (IPI) set the industry standard for improving athletic performance, showing athletes not only how to make dramatic gains in strength, explosion, flexibility, and power but also how to adapt that can-do mindset to other areas of their lives.

Nomar, who continued training with me while I was at IPI and when I moved to Arizona to build Athletes' Performance in 1999, used the program to add power, flexibility, and endurance. He put on 35 pounds of lean mass over a 5-year period, transforming from a skinny infielder with little power into an all-around player who could hit home runs. Not only that, he improved his agility so that he could become an even better fielder at shortstop, the most demanding position on the field.

Mary Pierce used the program to develop the power needed to compete in the modern world of women's tennis, capturing the 2000 French Open. Meghann Shaughnessy, another client, has risen as high as number 12 in the Women's Tennis Association rankings since joining our program.

Golfer Billy Mayfair thought chronic back problems would force him to retire in his early thirties. Instead, he's used our program to develop a more flexible, elastic body, one that's resistant to injury. He now talks about eventually playing on the Champions (formerly Senior) PGA Tour.

Nikolai Khabibulin, one of the top goalies in the National Hockey League, has used our program to keep his body elastic and stable, avoiding the groin and hamstring injuries so common to his position.

Our program also has helped dozens of athletes prepare for the National Football League's scouting combine, the testing ground for the NFL draft. Players such as Kyle Turley, Leonard Davis, and Levi Jones dramatically improved their strength, speed, power, and flexibility prior to the draft. As a result, they were picked higher and earned millions more in signing bonuses.

These players are specifically training to become faster, quicker, and stronger. Some are also trying to put on solid weight to compete in the NFL, where the majority of the players weigh between 240 and 340 pounds. Some need to go the opposite direction—to lose fat and get leaner.

We've even had some who come to our

program and say, "If only you could make me taller."

Technically, that should be impossible. But we've had instances in which athletes have literally measured ½ to 1 inch taller because their training enabled them to release and open up their hips, elongate their muscles, and restore their optimal alignment. They've been able to retract and depress their shoulder blades, which is to say they've pulled their scapulae back and down, extending the neck and head and, more important, stabilizing the body.

This isn't a problem that only athletes suffer. Most people are a little hunched over from the effects of gravity and spending too much time sitting, especially at a computer. As people age, they tend to lose an inch or two of height as their bodies slowly curl inward from the shoulders and neck. So it's probably happening to you.

If you've ever had a professional sports massage, you've noticed the tremendous relief that comes with releasing the tightness in your shoulder muscles and restoring your body's natural alignment. You probably didn't notice if the massage also made you a bit taller, although it very well could have.

With this program, you get that same effect, the release of tight muscles and the return to optimal alignment. I'm not going to promise you additional height, though you could enjoy a modest gain. I am confident, however, that you will feel taller and possibly even

appear taller to your acquaintances. That's because people who follow our program develop a confidence and energy level that friends notice. They may not be able to pinpoint the change, but they know it's there, sort of like when someone gets a new hairstyle or ditches her eyeglasses in favor of contact lenses or laser surgery.

Me, I'm an even 6 feet tall. But people tell me I seem taller because this program has given me perfect posture. When my coauthor and I attended some business meetings related to this book, Pete looked at my shoes, as if I were wearing lifts. I told him his frame of reference was off. Up until that point, he had seen me only at Athletes' Performance, where I look small compared to some of our clients.

Pete shook his head. Some of the people we were meeting with were taller than I am. But they tended to have that hunched-over, worn-down look typical of many Americans who work too much and exercise too little. I've been able to maximize my posture and alignment and create the illusion that I'm taller than I am.

As this program has evolved since its beginning 15 years ago, I've been guided by two underlying principles. First, everything needed to be geared toward making the body function better, not just for competitive athletes but also for people dealing with the demands of everyday life, especially as they age. Second, I realized that most people have limited time to take care of themselves physically, which is why I created this "greatest hits" version of the more extended programs we use at Athletes' Performance.

I first implemented what I now call the Core Workout with college athletes, who face a time crunch given the demands of classes, practice, and travel. I designed the program to derive the most benefit from the least amount of time.

Since your schedule is probably even more demanding than that of a college athlete, I've streamlined the process further to enable you to get the most out of your exercise in the same amount of time you're probably already dedicating to training.

We tend to think of athletes as people who excel in sports, but it's really more of a mindset common to people who want to improve, no matter the field or endeavor. We all have goals and want to improve, but we need the discipline and guidance to achieve those dreams.

This book provides that guidance. Think of it as the cheese and pickles that you've been missing.

CORE SELF-EVALUATION

Everyone who comes to train at Athletes' Performance undergoes a self-evaluation, assigning a rating of 1 to 5 in numerous areas, including balance, eye-hand coordination, flexibility, body weight, body composition, strength, resistance to injury, and resistance to illness. This process will give you a benchmark to measure improvement later.

Please take a few minutes right now to rate yourself in the following categories on a scale of 1 to 5 (1 = poor; 2 = fair; 3 = average; 4 = good; 5 = excellent).

Quality of sleep	1	2	3	4	5
Resistance to injury	1	2	3	4	5
Resistance to illness	1	2	3	4	5
Training knowledge	1	2	3	4	5
Nutritional knowledge	1	2	3	4	5
Motivation/desire	1	2	3	4	5
Past dedication to training	1	2	3	4	5
Overall healthy lifestyle	1	2	3	4	5
Mobility/flexibility	1	2	3	4	5
Muscle and joint tightness/pain (1 = lots; 5 = none)	1	2	3	4	5
Body composition (1 = unacceptably flabby; 5 = very lean)	1	2	3	4	5
Body weight (1 = very far from your target weight, no matter if you're under or over it; 5 = right at your target weight)	1	2	3	4	5
Strength	1	2	3	4	5
Endurance	1	2	3	4	5
Core/pillar strength (1 = current or chronic problems with your lower back and/or shoulders; 5 = injury-free)	1	2	3	4	5
Linear speed	1	2	3	4	5
Agility	1	2	3	4	5
Balance	1	2	3	4	5

CHAPTER 3

THE CORE CHALLENGE

What would you think if I said that you just filled out that self-evaluation incorrectly? I don't mean that literally; I'm sure you followed the directions and circled the proper responses. It's just that you'll likely discover by following this program that your frame of reference was way off and you never would have reached your potential without making changes in your training and lifestyle.

Let's say that you gave yourself a "5" for balance. Maybe you ice-skate or perform martial arts or do gymnastics. You have a good feel for balance. And it's very possible that you deserve a "5" for balance. But I'm willing to bet that when you start performing the exercises in this program, you might not feel as balanced as you think you are.

I'm also willing to bet that after you've done this program for a few weeks, you're going to be more balanced than you ever thought you could be. You'll come to realize that the "5" you gave yourself during the self-evaluation probably should have been a "3." That, or you deserve a "7" for your improved balance based on what you thought was the original five-point scale.

People who have used my program tell me they're reaching levels they never thought possible. Even professional athletes, people who seem able to do anything and everything physically, tell me they're reaching new heights.

The problem with most workout programs is that you end up hitting a wall quickly. You fall into a workout rut, doing the same exercises and failing to challenge your body further. So many people limit themselves before they even begin. They think they can be only so flexible or so strong or so fast. People are very good at perfecting the art of being average.

Since you've just signed your pledge of maximum performance, I know you're committed to reaching those new heights. So please don't tell me you're incapable. My biggest pet peeve is hearing, "I can't." Show me what you *can* do instead.

I'm going to show you how much of traditional training is inefficient and why many people only begin to tap into the full potential of their bodies. I'm going to explain the science and philosophies behind this program. I'm going to give you a better understanding of how your body works and how you can best train it for improved performance.

I'll break down your body into easy-to-understand components and focus on pillar strength, which comes from the dozens of muscles attached to the hips, pelvis, lower back, abdominals, ribs, and shoulder blades. These core muscles—though ignored by many trainers and athletes who focus on the biceps, triceps, and quadriceps—are the keys to all athletic movements. Not only that, they stabilize the body and improve its resistance to injury and long-term ailments. Your body moves in three dimensions, across three physical planes, but conventional weight training and cardio work each address only one dimension.

THE THREE PLANES OF MOTION

Imagine dividing your body from the top of your head straight down through your nose to the bottom so that you have left and right sides. This is the *sagittal* plane, which covers flexing and extending movements. Now imagine cutting straight across your waist so that you have a top and a bottom. This is the *transverse* plane, which covers rotational movements. Now imagine dividing yourself in half so that you were left with a front and a back. This is the *frontal* plane. In *Core Performance,* we're going to work across all three planes, often within the same movement, since movement is rarely one- or two-dimensional. During sports activities, for example, your body will move in all three planes.

It's vital to train for functional movement, not simply for the aesthetic benefit of having more muscle and less fat. We're not born with an obsession with our appearance. Rather, we have an inherent desire to master movements, experience freedom, and live fully. In this program, I want you to rediscover your inner toddler, the part of you that can't wait to master new movement skills.

Traditional training—from stretching to weight lifting to cardio work—doesn't begin to address the body's needs for joint support, endurance, and new challenges. The body can be trained to be more explosive, flexible, elastic, and functional in the same amount of time that many people already spend just to look better in front of a mirror. Even if you've trained for years, following all the latest exercise trends, I'll bet you've never rekindled that childhood joy of experiencing movement or tapped into this powerful sports science. As a result, you're probably training ineffectively and perhaps ignoring movements, body parts, and joints that are vital to your quality of life, let alone peak athletic performance.

I'm not going to overload you with a lot of technical jargon. But I do want you to have a better understanding of the reasoning behind what you'll do in the next section, the Core Workout.

BUILDING A SMARTER BODY

Most people take a passive approach to working out. Coaches and gym teachers tell you what to do at a young age. Adults hire personal trainers so they don't have to think too much about what they're doing. At most, you know that you're working out to lose weight, become leaner, or both.

Knowledge is empowering. I want you to understand the science behind what we're doing. I want you to realize that there's no reason to burden yourself with limitations based on what you've done in the past. You'll find, as all of our athletes have, that you will need to reevaluate your self-evaluation.

My ultimate goal is for you to understand this system so you can begin to enjoy the benefits and freedoms of this increased physical activity, regardless of your time commitments and workout facilities.

I want you to view this program as a means to transform not only your body but also your life. Throughout this book, I've included philosophies that have guided me in everything I do. I call them "core life principles." You'll also hear from professionals who have trained at Athletes' Performance. They'll tell you how they've taken the philosophies from the Core Workout and applied them to every aspect of their lives.

Near the end of the book, we'll talk specifically about applying these core life principles so that you can reach your goals and fulfill your dreams, no matter how far off and unimaginable they might seem today.

SETTING GOALS

The problem with many workout regimens is that people don't raise the bar high enough. Instead of setting specific goals, they come up with something ambiguous like "losing a few pounds" or "getting in better shape" or "firming up my belly."

Don't get me wrong; those are worthy aspirations, and you'll achieve them through this plan. But I've found that if people don't set specific goals, they don't maximize their results. Once they lose a few pounds or get in (slightly) better shape or drop an inch or two from the midsection, it's easy to rationalize missing a workout. After all, they've already reached those modest goals.

This also speaks to the issue of time. Everyone struggles to find enough time to work out. But what if you had more defined goals to

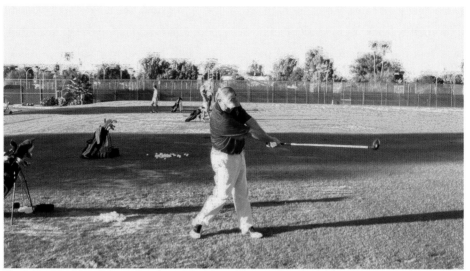

Scott Merrill, pictured above, is a financial advisor. After a serious back injury 3 years ago, he used our program not only to recover and strengthen his back but also to improve his recreational golf game by adding 20 yards to his drive.

serve as motivation, not just physical goals but *performance* goals?

For instance, do you play golf? What if I told you this program could add 20 yards to your drive? Do you participate in 5-K or 10-K races? What if you could shave minutes off your times? Do you play tennis? What if you could add a few miles per hour to your serve? What if you could dunk a basketball?

One of my senior athletes, a remarkable entrepreneur named T. C. Swartz, has never played professional golf but nonetheless is striving to join the Champions (formerly Senior) PGA Tour.

Maybe you don't play sports. I can appreciate that, though I would suggest that you're missing out on a great opportunity to spend time with friends, experience competition, and enjoy life. Even if you're not into sports, you probably have family members who are. Join them or use that time to do your own physical activity.

Maybe you'd like to play a sport but can't because of a physical ailment or lack of fitness. Your goal could be to get back into the game or compete in that sport for the first time. Would you like to run a marathon? That could be a specific goal.

Perhaps there's a quality-of-life area to address. My coauthor Pete Williams, who had back problems, set a goal of being able to drive 3 hours without having to get out of the car and stretch. Golfer Billy Mayfair wanted to avoid back surgery. Maybe you have an area of the body that's causing you trouble. Set a specific goal of regaining your physical abilities.

Take a moment right now and set five performance goals for yourself. Aim high and be as specific as possible. Studies show that people who put their goals in writing are far more likely to achieve them. I've placed a time frame on each of them so that you can achieve both short-term and long-term goals.

Goal One (3 months):

_____

_____

Goal Two (6 months):

_____

_____

Goal Three (1 year):

_____

_____

Goal Four (18 months):

_____

_____

Goal Five (2 years):

_____

_____

Now that you have a well-defined set of goals, let's embark on the Core Workout.

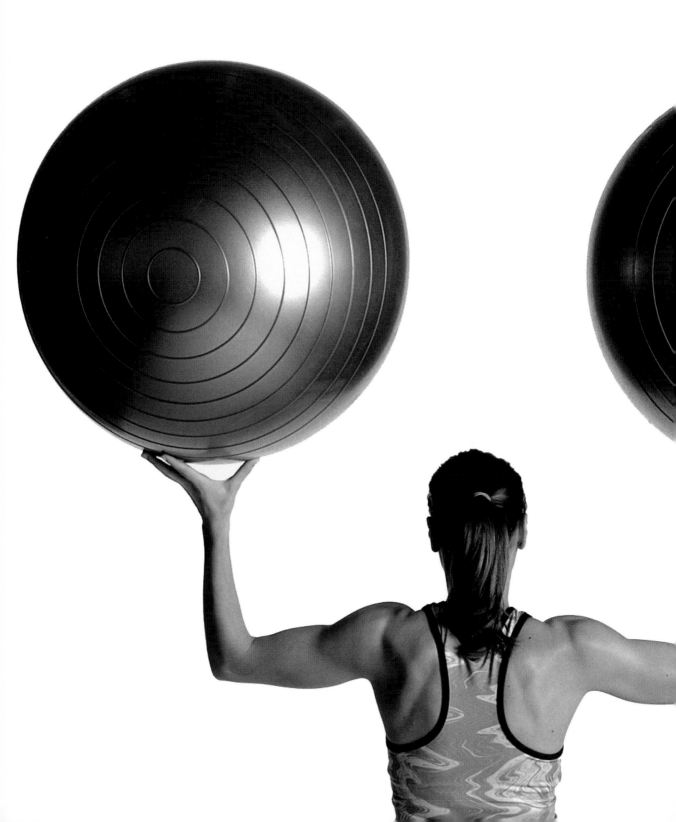

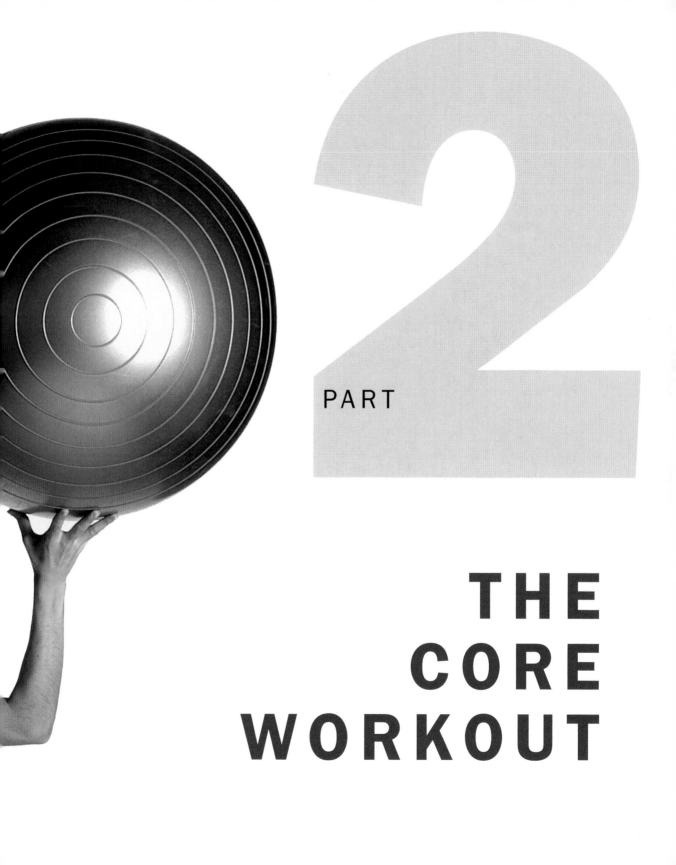

PART

2

THE CORE WORKOUT

CHAPTER 4

THE FOUNDATION: BUILDING YOUR PILLAR OF STRENGTH

We have a tendency to think of movement as starting from the limbs. If we reach out to grab something or step forward, we think of those motions as originating with the end result—we've reached out; therefore, we've used our arms. We've stepped forward, so we've worked our legs. Uncountable exercise programs promise bigger arms or sexier legs as a primary benefit.

Movement, however, starts from the very center of the body, the core area of the torso. Amputees still can function and have fulfilling lives because their cores remain intact. Frostbite begins at the fingers and toes, areas farthest from the core, because the body wants to protect what's most important and concentrates its lifesaving heat around the vital organs at the center of the body.

That's why we refer to the torso as the pillar—it's the structural center of movement and life. The way we maintain that pillar and its alignment and function directly correlate to the health of our organs and the rest of our bodies. Everything is interrelated.

Pillar strength, thus, is the foundation of movement. More specifically, it consists of core, hip, and shoulder stability. Those three areas give us a center axis from which to move. If you think of the body as a wheel, the pillar is the hub, and the limbs, the spokes.

We want to have the hub perfectly aligned so we can draw energy from it and effectively transfer energy throughout the body. It's impossible to move the limbs efficiently and with

PERFECT POSTURE ∎

Perfect posture is the proper stance for optimal movement. Your shoulder blades should be pulled back and down, and your tummy should be drawn up and in. If you're standing with perfect posture, your ears should be in line with your shoulders, your hips with your knees, and your knees with your ankles. If you're seated, there should be a line between your ears and hips.

force if they're not attached to something solid and stable.

The better you can transfer energy through your body, the more efficiently you will move, and the less wear and tear there will be. If you have good pillar strength and take a step, force will pass evenly through your foot, calf, and hip—right up the pillar and through the top of your head.

If you lack pillar strength, specifically hip stability, the energy "leaks out" at the hip, and the body must compensate. More pressure is placed down toward the knees and up toward the lower back, which over time can cause degenerative problems.

Parents are always telling their children to sit or stand up straight. There's a reason for that. Without pillar strength, without what I call *perfect posture,* you will significantly increase the potential for injury in a chain that starts with your lower back, descends all the way to your knees and ankles, and rises up to your shoulders and elbows.

Everything in your body is connected and related through this pillar of strength. Your shoulders and spine are related to the core

and gluteus maximus (or glutes), and they're interwoven in cross patterns that need to be tuned for maximum efficiency.

Think of a rubber band wrapped around your body. If one end is not attached, you will not develop enough tension. The band is fine, but unless both ends are attached solidly, there's no way to store, release, and transfer energy throughout your body.

For every action, there's a reaction. If I fire and move one muscle, it causes another muscle to react. The muscles stretch and snap back. This dynamic, multiplanar transfer of energy from front to back, side to side, and top to bottom creates fluid movement for people with the greatest pillar strength.

Marion Jones, the world-class sprinter, has tremendous pillar strength. As she sprints 100 meters, there's a smooth transfer of energy through her stable pillar that allows her to run at such great speed. There's perfect harmony between coordination, muscular strength, stability, balance, elasticity, and flexibility.

All movement starts from a remarkable muscle called the *transverse abdominis.* Think of the TA as nature's weight belt. It originates from the lower spine and wraps around and attaches to the ribs, abdominals, and pelvis. When we draw the belly button in toward the spine and up toward the ribs, we're essentially tightening a belt, ensuring the protection of the pelvis and lower back. Your natural weight belt stabilizes the pelvis and supports the torso.

Whenever movement begins, the TA is the first muscle that fires—or, at least, it should be. For many people, that ability is lost over time on account of injuries or sedentary lifestyles. We spend so much time in front of computers and televisions that we develop bad posture. Injuries are a result and exacerbate the problem further.

Workers at home-improvement stores are required to wear snug belts around their backs and abdominals when lifting or moving objects for safety reasons. They need to wear such devices because their bodies no longer activate their natural weight belts.

If we can learn (or relearn) how to activate the TA, we can rely on nature's weight belt and not wear additional support. We'll be able to stabilize the pelvis so that the leg and torso muscles can turn to it for support. That, in turn, prevents back problems. The body will be able to transfer force efficiently through the muscles rather than through the back and joints.

You'll relearn how to activate your TA early in this program, and though it's an easy process, you'll have to make a conscious effort at the beginning. Soon you'll find that it's second nature, and you will no longer have to think about it.

Now that you are conscious of the role of the transverse abdominis in core stability, we need to address your shoulders, another key element of perfect posture. Think of a skeleton hanging in a classroom. Its shoulders are naturally hanging back and down, giving it perfect posture and alignment.

Unfortunately, most people have a tendency to slump forward, with their shoulder blades sliding forward and up. If you spend much of your day in front of a computer, as many working Americans do, you're probably slumping over, even if you're not conscious of it. Unless you make some changes, you're going to end up hunched over like so many of our elderly friends who, sadly, never were exposed to a program like this years ago, when they most needed it.

I want you to keep your shoulder blades pulled back and down toward your waist, as if thrusting your chest up. You'll hear me reiterate it ("SBD") during the instructions for many exercises. It's important to keep your shoulders in this position throughout the program and throughout life.

Another key concept to understand about pillar strength is the *fascial* planes that wrap around the body. Think of these planes as the ropes that tie your muscles together. They ulti-

ACTIVATING THE TRANSVERSE ABDOMINIS ■

If I told you to get your tummy tight, chances are you would hold your breath as if preparing to be punched in the stomach. Or you'd get in an abdominal-crunch position, which, incidentally, is poor posture and puts needless stress on the back.

Instead, we want to think about maintaining perfect posture. Your abdominals are drawn in, but you're still able to breathe. If you waded into ice-cold water, you'd instantly stand up straight with your hips tall in order to keep as much of your body above the water line as possible. You would automatically pull your tummy in, activating the TA. I don't want you to have to do that, although I will explain the benefits of "cold plunging" later in the book.

For now, here are three popular ways to practice activating your transverse abdominis.

- While wearing a belt and without holding your breath, slightly pull your belly button away from the belt.
- While lying supine (on your back), imagine a hockey puck sitting atop your belly button. Move it up and down. (My colleague Michael Boyle has all of his pro hockey clients do this.)
- While lying supine, try to pull your belly button to your spine without holding your breath.

If you've gone through childbirth, the TA is the muscle from which you generated the force to push the baby out. (Thankfully, there are easier ways to activate the TA!)

COACHING KEY: Don't confuse the TA with the muscles of the pelvic floor, which are used to quit urinating. The pelvic muscles are important and work in conjunction with the TA to give you great stability.

In the early days of the Core Workout, you might find it useful to practice activating your TA while sitting at a desk or standing in front of a mirror as you shave or apply makeup. Be conscious of pushing out and sucking up and in. Make a conscious effort to keep your tummy tight throughout the 12-week program. If you do, you'll have much more success with turning your body into a pillar of strength.

---

mately tie a glute into your opposite shoulder and your hip muscles to your lower back.

Let's say you were standing on an observation deck looking directly down upon golfer Tiger Woods at the tee. As his club comes back, his shoulders turn, and his lower body remains stable, if only for a moment. At that instant, from your vantage point, his body would form the letter *X*. He's able to disassociate his shoulders and hips as he moves across the transverse plane to generate incredible power. Why? Because he's developed incredible mobility and pillar strength.

Tiger moves powerfully in three dimensions and so will you, once you've developed pillar strength. We're going to focus on the pillar in everything we do, which I bet is the opposite of how you're accustomed to working out.

You've probably been "training legs" or "working arms" on alternate days, perhaps with some ab work thrown in, time permitting. One of your goals might have been to develop a tight "six-pack" of abs.

I'm sure your intentions were good and your work ethic was sound. But focusing on arms, legs, and abs without integrating the pillar is like installing landscaping before building the house. Or buying an expensive set of wheels and tires for a car with a bent, rusted-out frame.

Starting with the next page, we're going to build the house first, making sure our foundation is strong. Don't get me wrong; you'll end up with nice abs. But they won't be the end goal, just one of many signs of your pillar of strength. So let's get started now by diving into the seven units of the Core Workout.

THE SUPER SEVEN

The Core Workout consists of the following seven units.

1. Movement Prep: an active warmup routine that replaces traditional pre-exercise stretching.

2. Prehab: a proactive approach to protecting yourself from injury.

3. Physioball Routine: a series of exercises to improve hip, core, and shoulder strength and stability.

4. Elasticity: a unit to help the body gen-erate force and make it springy, much like a pogo stick.

5. Strength: a new approach to resistance training based on training body *movements* for increased power, stability, and mobility.

6. Energy System Development (ESD): a departure from traditional cardio work, creating powerful bursts of energy.

7. Regeneration: a series of low-intensity activities designed to enhance recovery.

Exercises from each of these units will be organized into a 6-day-a-week workout, though I'll provide abbreviated versions for people traveling or crunched for time, along with 3-day versions for those people easing their way into the program. We'll train hard on 4 days (Monday, Tuesday, Thursday, and Friday) and devote Wednesday and Saturday to lighter Regeneration activities. You can tweak the days if you like, so long as you follow each 2-day period of intense training with a day of Regeneration.

Before we get to the details of these exercises and how they're organized, it's important to remember the need to maintain perfect posture and also an *athletic position.*

An athletic position is perfect posture with the legs slightly bent, the hips back, and the weight on the middle to front part of the foot. Take a few moments now to practice perfect posture and the athletic position.

Now you're ready for the first of our seven units: Movement Prep.

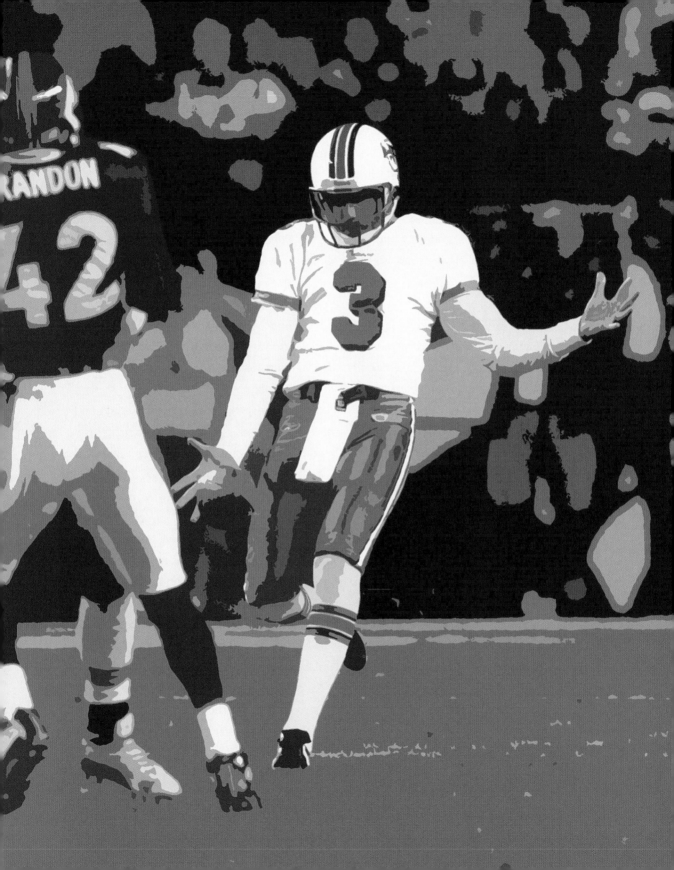

CHAPTER 5

MOVEMENT PREP

I f you've had any experience in sports or training, you've probably done some stretching. We're told from a young age that we need to stretch in order to prevent injury. Stretching is viewed as a precursor to working out, just as brushing your teeth is a precursor to going to bed. Not surprisingly, most people approach stretching routines halfheartedly.

There's tremendous value in traditional stretch-and-hold, or "static," stretching if executed properly, and it's part of the Core Workout—but only when done *after* a workout. After all, a warm rubber band stretches a lot farther than a cold one, right? So it's best to stretch when the body is warm, which it is after training. (We'll touch more on this in the Regeneration section of the workout.)

We've replaced preworkout static stretching with a Movement Preparation series of exercises that's an essential part of your routine, not just a necessary evil like stretching. In fact, if you were to incorporate just one element of this book into your existing workout routine, I'd want it to be Movement Prep. Nothing else provides so much value in so little time.

Movement Prep, as the term suggests, prepares the body for movement. It boosts heart rate, blood flow to the muscles, and core temperature. It also improves the function of the nervous system.

Think of the Movement Prep routine as taking a few minutes to warm up a car that has been sitting outside in cold temperatures all night. It also can be compared to a pilot's turning on all the switches in the cockpit before a flight. If you go through this checklist, you'll be dialed in physically and mentally for the rest of your workout. The end result will be a significant improvement in mobility, flexibility, and stability, on top of an increase of speed and power output by nearly 20 percent compared to static stretching.

CORE LIFE PRINCIPLE: MOVEMENT PREP

Just as a lack of physical movement is the biggest enemy to the body, a lack of movement and progress in other areas is the largest obstacle to a fulfilling life. We all have skills that we need to activate and use every day; otherwise, we lose them. We also wear multiple hats as child, parent, sibling, and friend, and must nurture these relationships daily; we can't take them for granted. Be proactive with everything you do. Don't just wait for things to happen. Activate and exercise your gifts and talents each day. No matter what you do, move forward!

CORE LIFE ACTION: What can you do right now to nurture a relationship? Make a phone call. Send an e-mail. Schedule some quality time right now.

We want to improve the long-term mobility and flexibility of muscles. Rather than have them stretch and go back to where they were—as is the case with traditional stretching—we want your body to remember those ranges of motion.

We do this through a process of lengthening the muscle (known as active elongation), which is no different from a traditional stretch. But then comes the crucial difference: After you stretch the muscle to this new range of motion, you contract the muscle. In other words, you don't just stretch the muscle and then end the stretch. You actually use it in that stretched position.

That does a couple of useful things. First, by strengthening muscles in that new range of motion, you stabilize all the tiny muscles around your joints that help hold the joints together. That will improve posture and performance and decrease the potential for injury. Second, and most important, we're going to "activate" these little muscles, throwing on the light switches so they're available and participating all the time.

Nearly all of the athletes we see for the first time have at least one muscle group that's completely shut off. This can cause other areas of the body to compensate, which ultimately leads to injury. An example of this would be one of the small muscles of the hips, the gluteus medius, which if not activated will lead to lower-back problems, knee pain, and groin strain. It's as if someone flipped the circuit breaker, cutting off the power to these little muscles.

And that's in elite athletes. Think of how many switches the average adult has deactivated, considering he rarely does anything more challenging than walking up or down stairs.

Thankfully, with Movement Prep, it takes only a day or two to reactivate these inactive areas. These 10 exercises, which require no equipment, enable your body to recall those movements that perhaps haven't been used since childhood. (If you are a young athlete, Movement Prep is going to make sure that you maintain the ability to perform these movements.)

Another difference between traditional stretching and Movement Prep is that the goal of the former is to relax muscles, to allow you to get into a stretched position and hold it. In Movement Prep, you're going to contract your muscles, which is to say you will be activating them by squeezing them.

Let's take your butt, which we prefer to call your gluteus maximus and usually shorten to "glutes." Take a moment and squeeze your left butt cheek, then your right. Pretty simple, right? Yet most people, even active athletes, rarely activate their glutes. As a result, they never take full advantage of these tremendously powerful muscles that should be a big part of everyday movement.

Instead, we spend most of our time sitting on our glutes, which causes the muscles opposite them—the hip flexors—to become tight and inactive. The neuromuscular relationship of these opposing muscle groups is known as *reciprocal inhibition,* which is a fancy way of saying that when one muscle group contracts, the other relaxes. When one fires, the other reloads. Movement Prep is reciprocal inhibition at work.

The Movement Prep routine wakes these muscles up—and not just for your workout. They'll remain switched on for the rest of the day. Here's why that's important: Let's say you're walking on a winter day, and your foot slips on some ice. How well your body reacts to that slip on the ice depends on your *proprioception,* the system of pressure sensors in the joints, muscles, and tendons that your body uses to maintain balance. Movement Prep, in switching on your body's small muscles, also tunes your sense of proprioception. It prepares your body for random, chaotic movement by fine-tuning its nerves and feedback mechanisms.

We'll generally do 5 to 10 repetitions of each of the Movement Prep exercises; not only will it feel like part of your workout (as opposed to a boring precursor to the real thing), at first it might feel like a workout itself. But don't worry: Your body will quickly condition itself to the exercises, and when you're done, you'll feel warmed up, rather than worn down. And you'll be better prepared for whatever follows, whether it's a workout, a game, or just the normal actions of everyday life.

SUMMARY: Movement Prep is going to increase your core temperature and elongate your muscles actively so that you make long-term flexibility gains. It will improve your balance and proprioception, and it is the perfect formula for building mobility, flexibility, stability, and strength.

TIME CAPSULE: Movement Prep requires no equipment and a minimum investment of time. I've provided different versions of the Core Workout to fit any lifestyle or level of training, but you'll find that Movement Prep is a common denominator. If you were to do nothing else, I would want you to commit to mastering and performing the Movement Prep routine two to six times a week, if only for 10 minutes. It provides a tremendous return for a minimum investment.

The following pages provide a look at the Movement Prep exercises. As with any new exercises, the pictures will help you better understand the movement. The selection and repetitions of each exercise will vary depending on the training goals for that particular day, week, and 3-week segment of the Core Workout, which are outlined in the full Core Workout worksheets (starting on page 176).

A CD-ROM featuring video of these exercises is available at www.coreperformance.com.

MARK ROYALS

NFL PUNTER
DATE OF BIRTH: 6/22/65

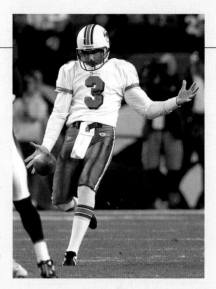

ON FLEXIBILITY AND MOVEMENT PREP

You might think that, as a 15-year veteran punter in the National Football League, I have incredible flexibility. Before I embarked on the Core Workout, I thought so, too. After all, I'm able to kick my right leg virtually as high as I want to generate the necessary loft and hang time on my punts.

As it turns out, I had one-dimensional flexibility—and only in my right leg at that. No wonder my left hip and lower back started to bother me when I reached my midthirties. If I wanted to keep playing, I had to try something different.

This program has opened me up to a whole new world of flexibility. Instead of performing a series of static stretches before games, I now go through the Movement Prep routine just like the one you're about to follow.

I've increased my flexibility, and my joints have become more stable as I've contracted through these new ranges of motion. I have greater proprioception, which is important when you're a punter and you have to get off a kick quickly and land safely with opponents (very, very big opponents!) coming at you.

Mark Verstegen has reaffirmed my belief that flexibility is vital, not just literally in sports but also metaphorically in life. I've played for six NFL teams, including two stints with the Tampa Bay Buccaneers, and my family and I have learned that it's important to be flexible, since my job can take us to another city at any time. Anyone who has been transferred around the country for work can relate to that.

When you move around that much, you learn that flexibility is essential as you try to fit into a new environment quickly. I've become an expert at that skill, to the point where I've usually been elected the player representative of my team. That's no small honor for a newcomer, let alone a punter, who isn't thought of as one of the traditional leaders in the locker room.

Flexibility is a key component of life because so many curveballs are thrown at you on a daily basis. If you're not flexible, you can create a lot of strife and hardship. For much of my career, I haven't known if I was going to have a job for the following season.

I've always had the flexibility to move elsewhere, but flexibility goes deeper than just playing in the NFL. If you have flexibility, you have the confidence to adapt to any situation, no matter how difficult.

Flexibility, as Mark is fond of saying, is about movement. And if you can master and perform the Movement Prep routine repeatedly, you'll soon develop the flexibility and mindset that you can handle anything.

HIP CROSSOVER

UNIT:
Movement Prep.

OBJECTIVE:
To build mobility and strength in your torso by disassociating hips and shoulders.

STARTING POSITION:
Lie supine (faceup) on the floor, arms and shoulders extended out at your sides and flat, feet flat on the floor.

PROCEDURE:
Twist your bent legs to the right until they reach the floor, then twist to the left.

COACHING KEY(S):
Keep your abs drawn in and shoulders, torso, and feet in contact with the ground.

YOU SHOULD FEEL:
Stretching and contracting of your core muscles.

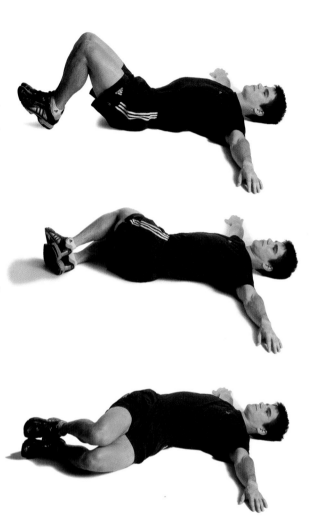

PROGRESSION:

Try this move with your hips and knees bent 90 degrees and your feet off the ground.

SECOND PROGRESSION:

Perform this move with your legs straight.

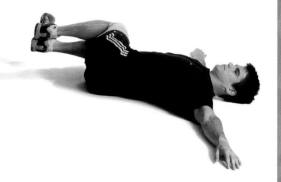

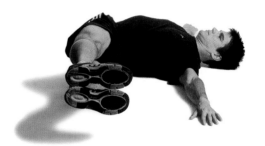

SCORPION

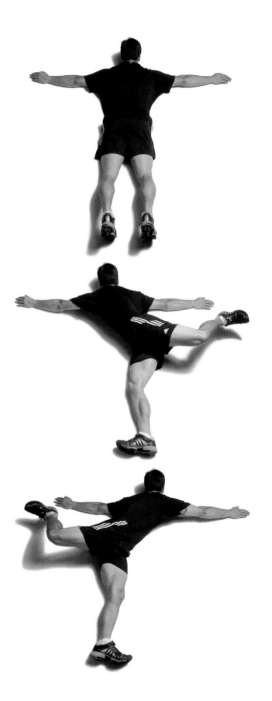

UNIT:
Movement Prep.

OBJECTIVE:
To lengthen and strengthen the muscles of your core; stretch your chest, quads, hips, and abs; and activate your glutes.

STARTING POSITION:
Lie prone (belly-down) on the floor, with your arms and shoulders pinned in the "spread 'em!" pose.

PROCEDURE:
Thrust your left heel toward your right hand by firing your left glute while keeping your right hip glued to the ground. Alternate legs.

COACHING KEY(S):
Be sure to fire (squeeze) your glute as you thrust your heel.

YOU SHOULD FEEL:
A stretch in your quads and hip flexors, along with activation of your glutes.

CALF STRETCH

UNIT:
Movement Prep.

OBJECTIVE:
To increase flexibility in this very often-neglected area.

STARTING POSITION:
From the pushup position, place your left foot over your right heel. Your weight should be on the ball of your right foot.

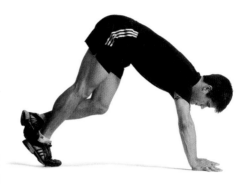

PROCEDURE:
Pull your right toes up toward your shin while you push your right heel down toward the ground with your left foot. Exhale as you lower your heel. Hold for a one count, raise your right heel again, and repeat.

COACHING KEY(S):
You're pulling your toes up toward the shin at the same time you're pushing the heel to the ground. Then push back through the new range of motion.

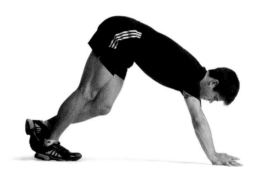

YOU SHOULD FEEL:
A stretch in your calf and ankle.

PROGRESSION:
Bend the knee of your working leg to shift the emphasis to your Achilles tendon.

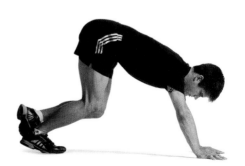

HAND WALK

A.k.a. "World's Second-Greatest Stretch"

UNIT:

Movement Prep.

OBJECTIVE:

To build stability in your shoulders and core and to lengthen your hamstrings, calves, and lower-back muscles.

STARTING POSITION:

Stand with your legs straight and hands on floor.

PROCEDURE:

Keeping your legs straight and belly button drawn in, walk your hands out. Still keeping your legs straight, walk your feet back up to your hands.

COACHING KEY(S):

Use short "ankle steps" to walk back up to your hands. That is, take baby steps using only your ankles—don't use your knees, hips, or quads.

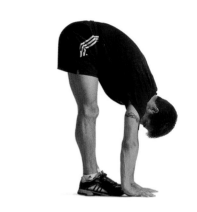

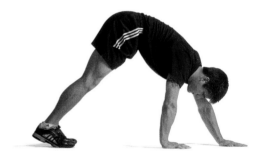

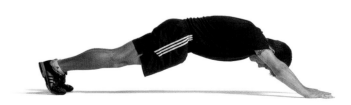

YOU SHOULD FEEL:

A stretch in your hamstrings, lower back, glutes, and calves and a burning in the fronts of your shins.

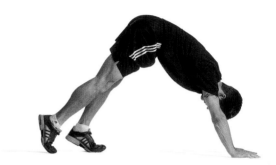

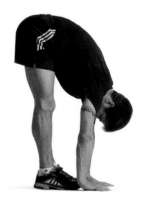

INVERTED HAMSTRING

UNIT:
Movement Prep.

OBJECTIVE:
To improve hamstring flexibility and balance, along with dynamic pillar stabilization.

STARTING POSITION:
Balance on your right foot with perfect posture (tummy tight, shoulders back and down).

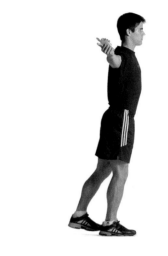

PROCEDURE:
Bending at the waist, and maintaining perfect posture, grab your right foot with your left hand, extending your left leg back as you fire the left glute. (You might find it easier to extend forward with both hands out, as shown, rather than while grabbing a foot.) Your shoulder and heel should move as one, forming a straight line. Take a step back at the end of each rep as you alternate legs.

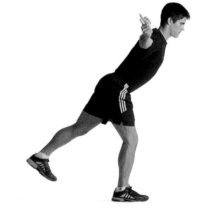

COACHING KEY(S):
Your body should be in a straight line from ear to ankle. Keep your back and pelvis flat! Someone should be able to place a broomstick snugly across your back.

YOU SHOULD FEEL:
A stretch in your hamstrings.

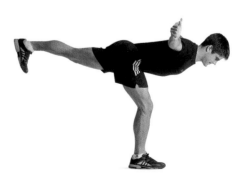

LATERAL LUNGE

UNIT:
Movement Prep.

OBJECTIVE:
To open up the muscles of your groin and hips. Also to hold pillar strength as you sit back and down.

STARTING POSITION:
Stand with perfect posture.

PROCEDURE:
Step out to the right, keeping your toes pointed straight ahead and feet flat. Squat by sitting back and down onto your right leg, keeping your left leg straight and the weight on the right leg's midfoot to heel. Squat as low as possible, keeping your left leg straight and holding this position for 2 seconds. Return to the standing position and repeat.

COACHING KEY(S):
Keep your feet pointed straight ahead and flat throughout.

YOU SHOULD FEEL:
A stretch in the inside of your thigh.

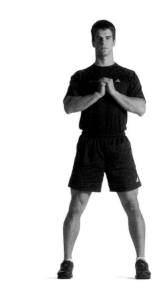

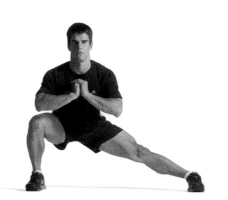

FORWARD LUNGE/
FOREARM-TO-INSTEP
A.k.a. "World's Greatest Stretch"

UNIT:
Movement Prep.

OBJECTIVE:
To improve flexibility in your hips, hamstrings, lower back, torso, groin, hip flexors, and quads.

STARTING POSITION:
Take a large step forward with your left leg, as if doing a lunge. Place and support weight on your right hand, even with your left foot.

PROCEDURE:
Take your left elbow and reach down to your instep (forward leg) while keeping your back knee off the ground. Then move your left hand outside your left foot and push your hips straight to the sky, pulling your toe up toward your shin. Finally, step forward into the next lunge.

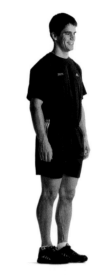

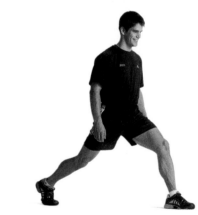

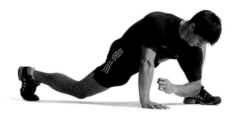

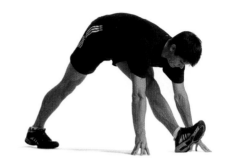

COACHING KEY(S):

Keep your back knee off the ground. Exhale as you reach your elbow to the floor. At the end, make sure both hands remain in contact with the ground as you lift your hips and pull your toe toward the shin.

YOU SHOULD FEEL:

A stretch in your groin, your back leg's hip flexor, and your front leg's glute. During the second part, you should feel a stretch in your front leg's hamstring and calf.

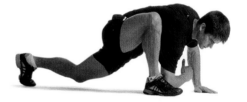

MOVEMENT PREP

BACKWARD LUNGE WITH A TWIST

UNIT:
Movement Prep.

OBJECTIVE:
To lengthen your hip flexors, quads, and core. This stretches everything from your big toes to your hands.

STARTING POSITION:
With your feet together, step back with your right leg into a lunge.

PROCEDURE:
Arch your back slightly while twisting your torso over your left leg and while reaching your right hand to the sky. Push back and out of that position into the next lunge.

COACHING KEY(S):
As you lean back and rotate, fire (squeeze) the glute of your back leg. This creates reciprocal inhibition, lengthening your hip flexors.

YOU SHOULD FEEL:
A stretch from your back leg through your core and lats, and a stretch of your hip flexors.

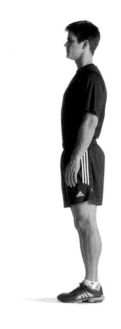

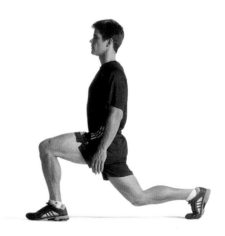

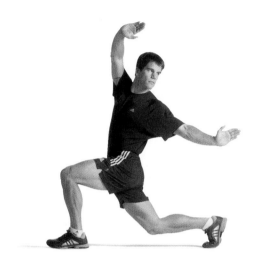

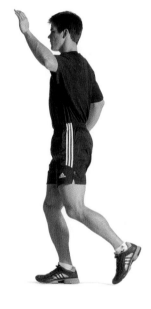

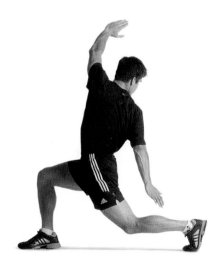

DROP LUNGE

UNIT:
Movement Prep.

OBJECTIVE:
To improve flexibility in your hips, glutes, and iliotibial (IT) bands—thick bands of tissue in either leg that extend from the thigh down over the outside of the knee and attach to the tibia (the larger lower-leg bone).

STARTING POSITION:
Stand balanced with your arms extended.

PROCEDURE:
Turn your hips to the left and reach back with your left foot until it's about 2 feet to the outside of your right foot, your left toes pointing to your right heel. Rotate your hips back so they're facing forward again and square with your shoulders and feet. You want your chest up and tummy tight, and the majority of your weight on your right leg. Drop into a full squat by pushing your hips back and down, keeping your right heel on the ground. Now drive hard off your right leg, stand back up, and repeat, moving to your right for the allotted number of reps. Switch legs. Return to the left.

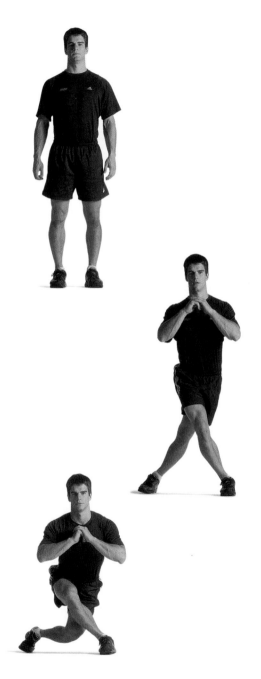

MOVEMENT PREP

COACHING KEY(S):

Turn your hips to drop your leg behind. Keep your toes pointed straight, with the back toe to the front heel.

YOU SHOULD FEEL:

A stretch in your hips, glutes, and IT bands.

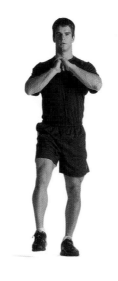

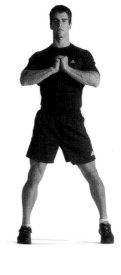

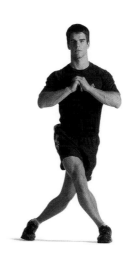

SUMO SQUAT-TO-STAND

UNIT:
Movement Prep.

OBJECTIVE:
To improve flexibility in your hamstrings, groin, ankles, and lower back.

STARTING POSITION:
Stand tall, with your feet outside your hips.

PROCEDURE:
Bend at the waist, grabbing under your big toes. Keeping your arms straight and inside your knees, pull your hips down until they're between your ankles, and lift your chest up. Then tuck your chin and try to straighten your legs, holding on to your toes as you straighten out your hips and knees.

COACHING KEY(S):
Hold on to your toes at the bottom of the movement. Pull your chest up and your shoulders back and down, and try to drive your hips forward to get your torso vertical, not horizontal. As you lift your hips, keep your back flat.

YOU SHOULD FEEL:
A stretch in your groin, glutes, lower back, and, to a lesser degree, ankles.

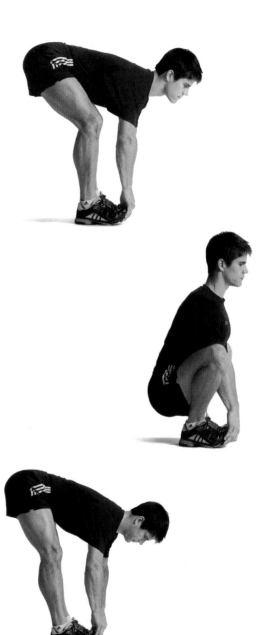

BRANDON WOOD

PROFESSIONAL BASEBALL PLAYER

DATE OF BIRTH: 3/2/85

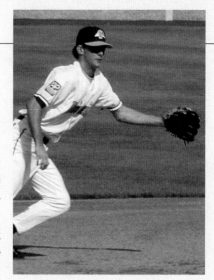

ON CORE PERFORMANCE *FOR YOUNG ATHLETES*

I began training with Mark Verstegen in 1999, when I was just 14. Though I had hoped the program would help make me a better high school baseball player, my main goal was simply to learn how to live a healthier life, since my family has a history of diabetes and heart disease.

When I started the program, I stood 5 feet 10 and weighed just 120 pounds. I dreamed of playing sports professionally, like so many other kids, but I didn't have the physical tools to do so. As a baseball player, I was a very good fielder but could barely hit the ball out of the infield because my body could not generate enough power.

Lots of kids have talent. The difference is that they don't know how to train for powerful movements and improve their core stability. They know little about proper nutrition. Many kids lift weights and run, but they don't have an integrated system that complements their sport-specific training.

Mark's program not only improved my physical performance but also gave me the confidence that I could achieve my biggest goals. Not long after I began training at Athletes' Performance, I set my sights on a college scholarship. Even that goal turned out not to be high enough.

Not only was I offered scholarships, I was selected in the first round of the Major League Baseball draft by the Anaheim Angels. Now, 4 years after I began this program, I'm on my way toward reaching my dream of playing in the major leagues. I never would have been in this position without Mark's program.

I was fortunate to live near Athletes' Performance in Tempe, Arizona. My parents had the means for me to train there, and Mark allowed me to work out at the facility. Not everyone can do that, of course, but with this book any kid can apply these same techniques to help fulfill his dreams if he's willing to make a commitment.

I'm now 6 feet 3 and weigh 185 pounds, which is still skinny by the standards of professional sports. I have a lot of work to do to reach the major leagues, and I'll continue to follow this program, not only throughout my pro career but afterward. I don't want to develop the health problems that have plagued my family. I'm confident that this program can take me to the highest levels imaginable, not just in sports but also in anything I want to achieve.

Four years ago, I was one of few kids who had access to this program. I considered it my secret weapon. It opened my eyes and showed me that I no longer had to be limited by my body. If you're a kid, make the commitment now to embrace this program and follow your dreams.

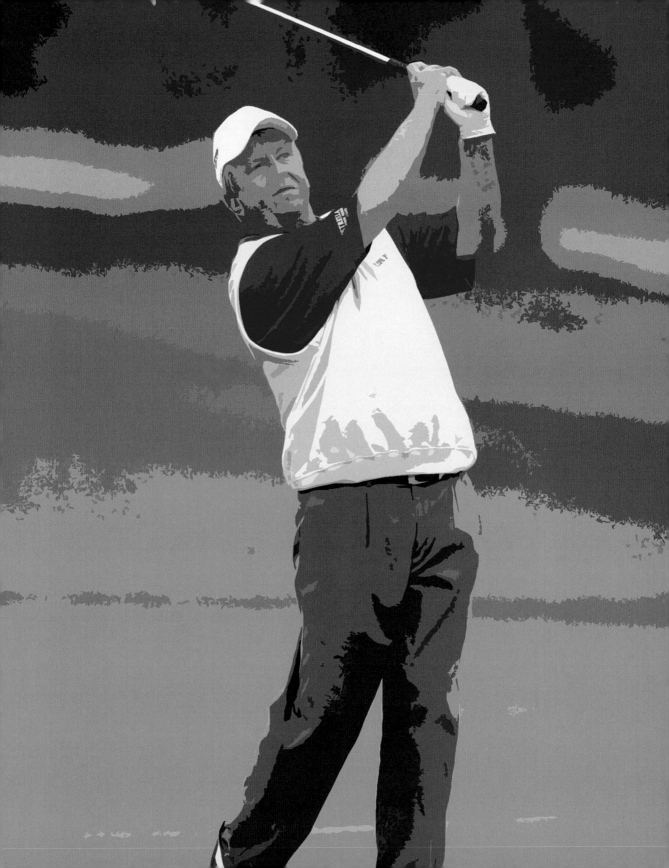

CHAPTER 6

PREHAB

Many years ago, people thought Honda was crazy when it asked auto buyers to bring their cars in for service every 3,000 miles. Why, they asked, would you take the car in when there's nothing wrong with it? These days, it's the norm to have a car checked out and to get an oil change every 3,000 miles.

No one has to ask why anymore. We all know that if you take care of a car, fewer things will go wrong with it. The same is true with your body. With the Prehab exercises in this chapter, we're going to strengthen the most vulnerable areas that get stressed in everyday movement: your hips, core, and shoulders. This is your pillar, and strengthening it will improve posture and alignment, allowing your joints to move more efficiently. It will also build up your most injury-prone areas before you're struck with chronic aches and pain that may, in the worst cases, require surgery.

Since the Core Workout is an integrated program, there's a degree of prehab in everything we do. But the Prehab unit is specifically geared toward strengthening the body to optimize mobility, balance, stability, and joint function and to decrease the potential for injuries while improving performance.

Moreover, Prehab helps correct problems created by your life outside the workout studio or playing field. You probably spend long hours hunched over a computer—most of us do. Inevitably, your shoulders roll forward and tighten. That's bad enough, but now let's say that you go out and try to play tennis. Since your shoulders are so tight, they lack the necessary stability and range of motion. Your body has a knack for compensating, however, and you end up using more of your elbows when you swing the racquet. That, combined with the poor joint alignment caused by your poor posture at work, could produce a nasty case of tennis elbow (or rotator cuff issues or upper-back spasms).

CORE LIFE PRINCIPLE: PREHAB

Just as a lack of prehabilitation will result in painful injuries and surgeries that will require rehabilitation, a lack of preparation in other areas of your life will result in painful developments later. If you don't take daily care of your body, relationships, career, and mental health, you're going end up in a situation requiring some major rehabilitation and damage control. By then, it could be too late. Apply prehab to all areas of your life, taking consistent action not only to prevent damage from neglect but also to educate yourself, develop strategies, and take daily steps toward reaching your goals. Be proactive, not reactive.

CORE LIFE ACTION: Take a moment right now and apply prehab to some area of your life to head off a downward spiral. Take action to remedy a troubling situation.

With Prehab, we're going to strengthen the muscles supporting your upper back and shoulder rotators. This improves your posture by pulling your shoulder blades back and down. The shoulder joint's ball and socket will move freely and efficiently, as it was designed to do. You will feel the difference in every aspect of your life.

Sitting at a desk all day also puts undue stress on your lower back and inevitably affects your core. After a long day on the job, it's difficult, if not potentially harmful, to go out and do something that requires strength in your torso without first "waking it up." So another goal of Prehab is to build core stability to protect your back from these daily stresses.

But the problems with modern life don't stop at your back. Lots of sitting also causes the hips to become locked down and less mo-bile. The hips support the pelvis and have more musculature attached to them than any other joints in the body. We want to make sure your hips have exceptional mobility and stability so that they can keep your pelvis in alignment. The Prehab exercises work on this area.

Here's how all this preemptive protection of your shoulders, lower back, and hips ultimately improves your life: About 65 percent of injuries—both athletic and lifestyle-related—come from overuse, which is to say from repetitive use of joints that are rendered dysfunctional by muscular imbalances. Since Prehab addresses the muscular imbalances that lead to the injuries, it helps prevent many lower-back injuries, shoulder-joint problems, and hamstring pulls, for instance.

The other 35 percent of injuries are caused by trauma, and we may as well be honest here:

If you run into a wall or take a tumble on the ski slope, something is likely to break, regardless of how carefully you've followed the Core Workout. Still, Prehab and the other units can improve your chances. Maybe, because of your balance and stability, you won't tumble at all. Maybe you'll tumble but not suffer as hard a fall as you would have before training. Professional skiers, for example, can walk away from nasty falls that would leave out-of-shape skiers paralyzed or even dead, because the pros have developed stability, elasticity, and strength. And even if you do fall and get hurt, your conditioned body should recover faster from the injury.

Once you've built pillar strength through the Prehab unit and the Physioball Routine in the next chapter, you've gone a long way toward creating a body that's capable of remarkable movement and, more important, is resistant to injury and long-term deterioration.

SUMMARY: Prehab is the proactive approach to protecting yourself from injury. Pillar strength, which consists of hip, shoulder, and core stability, is the foundation to efficient human movement and is vital to optimizing performance and health.

TIME CAPSULE: We'll perform the Prehab routine two to six times a week. Aside from the exercises involving a physioball, it requires no equipment. I want you to commit to spending at least 5 minutes a day on Prehab. You owe it to yourself to find the time—it's one of the best investments you can make in your long-term health.

A CD-ROM featuring video of these exercises is available at www.coreperformance.com.

BILLY MAYFAIR

PROFESSIONAL GOLFER

DATE OF BIRTH: 8/6/66

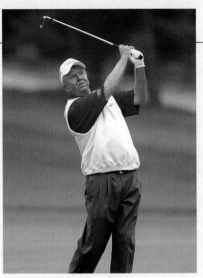

ON PREHAB AND QUALITY OF LIFE

A few years ago I tore fibers around disks in my lower back. Surgery was an option; prolonged rest, another. If my career wasn't in jeopardy, I certainly seemed unlikely to play at my best ever again.

By following the Core Workout, especially the Prehab portion, I was able to strengthen all the muscles around my back. It healed without surgery, and my game not only recovered, it improved. Instead of facing early retirement, I can look forward to a long PGA career and then join the Champions Tour.

The dangerous thing about golf is that we're always swinging in one direction. It's like lifting weights with only one arm. With the exception of left-handed golfers, most players have left sides far stronger than their rights. (Lefties, of course, have stronger right sides.) The beauty of this program, especially all the core-stability work, is that it evens out your body.

Not only that, it keeps your body loose. I sometimes hear recreational golfers talk about how it takes them nine holes to really get loosened up after working all day. Either that, or they have to spend time on the driving range beforehand. If you follow a program like this, you can loosen up on the first tee and get going.

A lot of people enjoy golf, but if you're in pain and out of shape, you can't play to your highest ability. You can pay $500 an hour for private lessons and $4,000 for custom-made clubs, but if your body isn't working in the right motion, you're going to struggle.

I've been on the PGA Tour for 13 years, and I've never felt stronger and more flexible. When your body feels good in the morning, it helps the way you play.

I relearned the proper way to bend down and pick up something off the ground, using not just my legs but also my glutes. I used to bend at the waist, which put tremendous strain on my back. Now I maintain perfect posture and squat using my hips, lifting with the big muscles of the legs rather than the small muscles in the back.

Like a lot of people with back pain, I lived with constant fear that I'd turn the wrong way and blow out my back. It affected not only my golf game but also my personal life. I worried that I wouldn't be able to pick up my son when he got to be 5 or 6 years old.

Now that I engage actively in prehab, I no longer have to worry about back problems. This program has helped my golf game, but I'm just as grateful that it's helped me be a better dad. And you don't have to be a professional golfer to appreciate that.

FLOOR/PHYSIOBALL Y

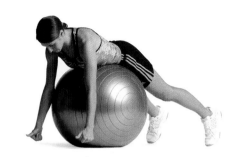

UNIT:

Prehab.

OBJECTIVE:

To improve shoulder stability, thus further strengthening your rotator cuffs. Also to improve scapular (shoulder blade) strength and muscle-recruitment patterns.

STARTING POSITION:

Lie prone (facedown) over the top of the ball so that your back is flat and your chest is off the ball.

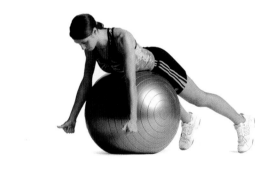

PROCEDURE:

While gliding your shoulder blades back and down toward your waist, lift your arms above your head to form a *Y*. Lower your chest and arms and repeat.

COACHING KEY(S):

Keep your thumbs up. Move from the scapulae (shoulder blades), extending your torso, shoulders, and hands. The top of your abs should be in the middle of the ball.

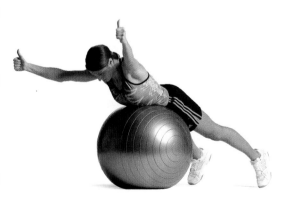

YOU SHOULD FEEL IT:

In your back, lower shoulder blades, and the fronts of your shoulders.

PROGRESSION:

Add weight, one pound at a time.

Note: If you're on the road or without a physioball, do the same exercise on the floor or on an exercise bench.

FLOOR/PHYSIOBALL *T*

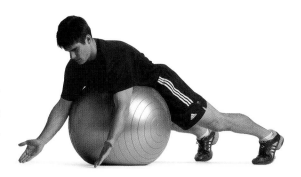

Prehab.

OBJECTIVE:

To improve shoulder stability, thus further strengthening your rotator cuffs. Also to improve scapular strength and muscle-recruitment patterns.

STARTING POSITION:

Lie prone over the top of the ball so that your back is flat and your chest is off the ball.

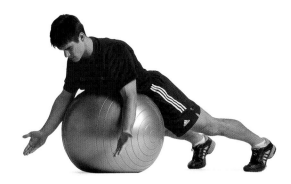

PROCEDURE:

Pull your shoulder blades in toward your spine and extend your arms to the sides to create a *T* with your torso. Keep your arms long and straight, 90 degrees to your torso. Your thumbs should be up and pointed toward the ceiling.

COACHING KEY(S):

Keep your head in line with your spine. Keep your shoulder blades back and down, trying to squeeze them together.

YOU SHOULD FEEL IT:

In the backs of your shoulders and in your upper back between the shoulder blades.

Note: If you're on the road or without a physioball, do the same exercise on the floor or on an exercise bench.

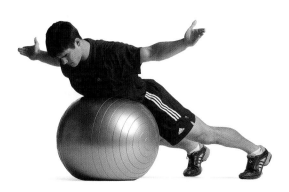

FLOOR/PHYSIOBALL *W*

UNIT:
Prehab.

OBJECTIVE:
To improve shoulder stability, thus further strengthening your rotator cuffs. Also to improve scapular strength and muscle-recruitment patterns.

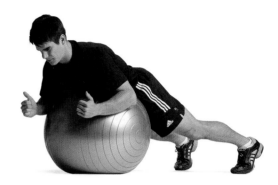

STARTING POSITION:
Lie prone over the top of the ball so that your back is flat and your chest is off the ball.

PROCEDURE:
Squeeze your elbows in toward your ribs. Take your thumbs and rotate them back toward the ceiling, squeezing your shoulder blades together to form a *W*. Continue to rotate your hands back as far as possible, keeping your elbows at your sides.

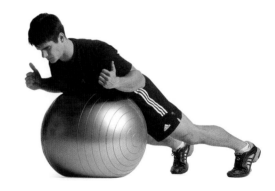

COACHING KEY(S):
Be sure to rotate your thumbs so that you feel the squeeze in your lower shoulder blades.

YOU SHOULD FEEL IT:
Deep in the posteriors (backs) of your shoulders.

Note: If you're on the road or without a physioball, do the same exercise on the floor or on an exercise bench.

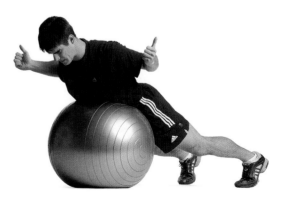

FLOOR/PHYSIOBALL *L*

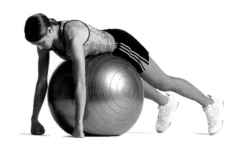

UNIT:

Prehab.

OBJECTIVE:

To improve shoulder stability, thus further strengthening your rotator cuffs. Also to improve scapular strength and muscle-recruitment patterns.

STARTING POSITION:

Lie prone over the top of the ball so that your back is flat and your chest is off the ball.

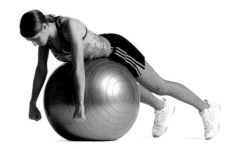

PROCEDURE:

Flex your elbow until it creates a 90-degree angle with your upper arm. Then squeeze your shoulder blades together to raise your upper arms so they're 90 degrees to your torso, creating a pair of *L*s. While holding that position, externally rotate your upper arms so that the backs of your hands reach toward the ceiling. Slowly retrace the pattern back to the starting position.

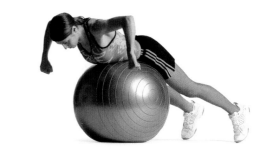

COACHING KEY(S):

Be sure to squeeze your shoulder blades, keeping your shoulders back and down. Rotate your hands back as far as possible.

YOU SHOULD FEEL IT:

Deep in the posteriors (backs) of the shoulders.

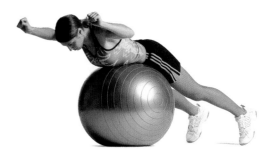

Note: If you're on the road or without a physioball, do the same exercise on an exercise bench or off the edge of your bed.

PHYSIOBALL PUSHUP PLUS

UNIT:

Prehab.

OBJECTIVE:

To improve core and shoulder stability. Also to increase strength in your shoulders, chest, and triceps.

STARTING POSITION:

Get in the pushup position, with your hands on the ball and your fingers pointed down the sides of the ball. Shoulder blades should be pushed away from each other in "plus" position (as far forward as possible).

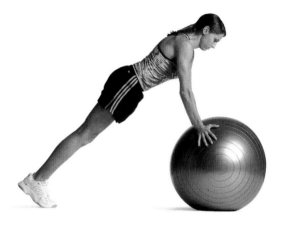

PROCEDURE:

With your belly button drawn in, lower yourself to where your chest barely grazes the ball. Control the ball as you push back up, holding your belly button in and protracting, or "plussing" out of, the shoulder blades to get as far away from the ball as possible.

COACHING KEY(S):

Lock your belly button in to stabilize your pillar before starting. Keep your body straight from ear to ankle.

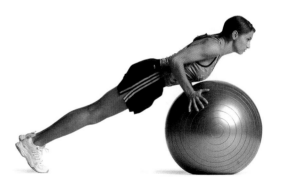

YOU SHOULD FEEL IT:

In your abs, chest, shoulders, and triceps.

GLUTE BRIDGE

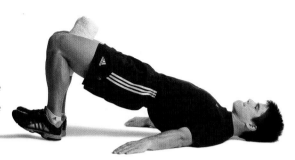

UNIT:
Prehab.

OBJECTIVE:
To activate, develop, and improve the firing/muscle-recruitment patterns of the glutes.

STARTING POSITION:
Lie supine (faceup) on the floor, with your knees bent 90 degrees and feet flat on the floor. Squeeze a rolled-up towel, a doubled-over TheraBand pad, or even a ball between your knees.

PROCEDURE:
With your belly button drawn in, bridge your hips toward the ceiling by firing your glutes. Only your shoulders and heels remain on the ground. Maintain a strong hip contraction throughout the range of motion. Hold, then lower your hips toward the floor without touching it and then repeat.

COACHING KEY(S):
Initiate the movement with your glutes, and don't let the glutes come all the way down.

YOU SHOULD FEEL IT:
In your glutes, not your lower back and hamstrings.

PROGRESSION:

When you've mastered that, try "marching" with one leg at a time.

SECOND PROGRESSION:

Try it with one leg straight and in line with your torso, and your weight supported on the other leg. Switch legs.

THIRD PROGRESSION:

Pull your left knee to your chest, then bridge off your opposite leg. Switch legs.

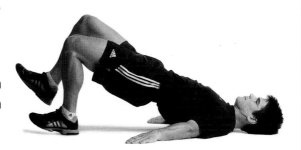

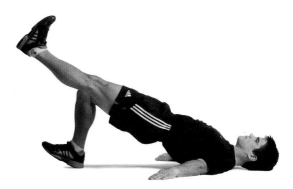

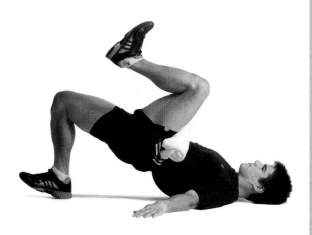

SIDE-LYING ADDUCTION AND ABDUCTION

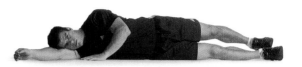

Prehab.

OBJECTIVE:
To activate and stabilize your hips.

STARTING POSITION:
Lie on your side, resting your head on your arm. Your legs should be straight out, with the top leg slightly behind your hips with your toes pointed ahead.

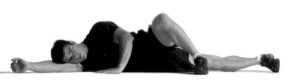

PROCEDURE:
Lift your top leg skyward. This is called *abduction.* For *adduction,* take the top foot and cross it over the bottom. Then lift your bottom leg by firing (squeezing) the inner muscles of that leg.

COACHING KEY(S):
Keep your belly button drawn in. When moving your top leg, fire the abductors, the muscles on the outside of your leg.

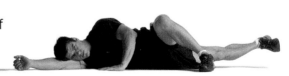

YOU SHOULD FEEL IT:
Above the hip joint at the inside part of your leg, between your hip and waist.

QUADRUPED CIRCLES

UNIT:
Prehab.

OBJECTIVE:
To stabilize your spine and create mobility, stability, and strength in your hips.

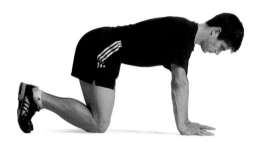

STARTING POSITION:
Set up on your hands and knees with your belly button drawn in and your shoulders protracted (extended, or pushed away from each other).

PROCEDURE:
Tuck your right knee to your chest. Fire the glute and lift the leg out to the side of your hip (think of a dog hosing down a fire hydrant), and rotate it in a circle until your leg is tucked back into your chest. Reverse the motion for the same number of reps and then repeat with your other leg.

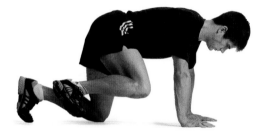

COACHING KEY(S):
Keep your belly button drawn in and your pelvis stable as you move your hip. This works the tiny stabilizer muscles between the vertebrae, called the multifidus, along with the muscles of the hip.

YOU SHOULD FEEL:
Your hips rotating.

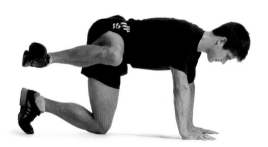

PILLAR BRIDGE FRONT

UNIT:
Prehab.

OBJECTIVE:
To create pillar (shoulder/core/hip) stability and strength.

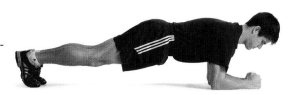

STARTING POSITION:
Lie facedown in a prone pushup position, with your forearms resting on the floor. Your elbows are under your shoulders and bent 90 degrees.

PROCEDURE:
Push up off your elbows, supporting your weight on your elbows. Tuck your chin so your head is in line with your body, and pull your toes toward your shins.

COACHING KEY(S):
Protract your shoulder blades while keeping your belly button drawn in. Keep your head in line with your spine—your body should form a straight line from ears to heels.

YOU SHOULD FEEL IT:
In your shoulders and core.

PROGRESSION:

Lift one arm or leg, hold for 2 seconds.
Switch arms or legs.

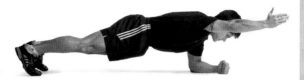

SECOND PROGRESSION:

Alternate opposites. Lift right arm and left
leg. Switch, lifting left arm and right leg.

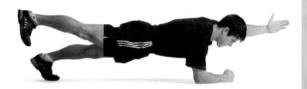

PILLAR BRIDGE SIDE, RIGHT AND LEFT

UNIT:
Prehab.

OBJECTIVE:
To create pillar (shoulder/core/hip) stability and strength.

STARTING POSITION:
Lie on your side with your forearm on the ground and your elbow under your shoulder. Your body should be in a straight line with your toes pulled toward your shins.

PROCEDURE:
Push up off your elbow, creating a straight line from your ankle to your shoulder.

COACHING KEY(S):
Be sure to push your hips off the ground and keep your toes up. Only the side edge of your bottom foot and your elbow should be in contact with the ground. Keep your hips pushed forward and body straight. Don't sag or bend!

YOU SHOULD FEEL IT:
In your hips, core, and shoulders, along with your bottom-side glute and obliques (the abdominal muscles on the side of your waist).

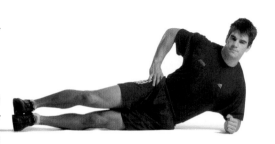

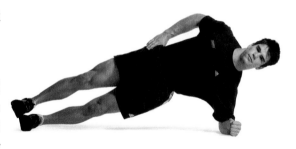

PROGRESSION:

Hold for 20 seconds. If this is too hard, do 10 reps of 2 seconds each.

SECOND PROGRESSION:

From the bridge position, lift your top leg as if performing a lateral jumping jack.

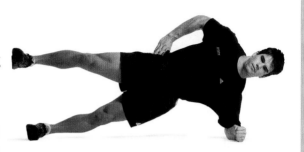

THIRD PROGRESSION:

Tuck your bottom leg into your chest and hold. You should feel it in the groin area of your top leg.

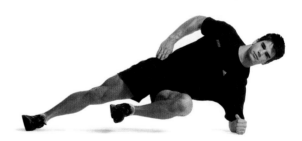

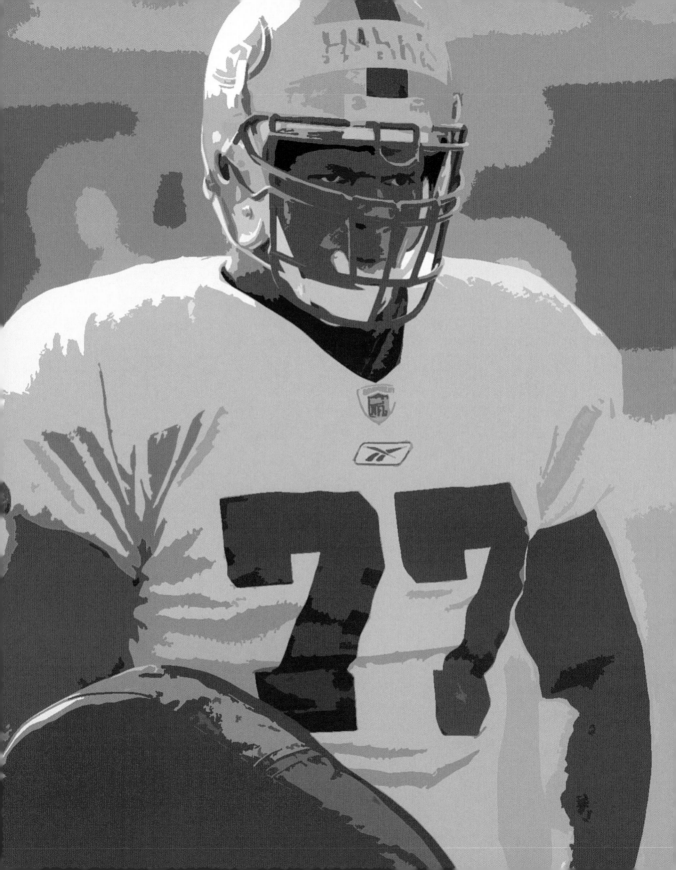

CHAPTER 7

PHYSIOBALL ROUTINE

The physioball (also called a Swiss, stability, or balance ball) is a simple device, but one of the most important pieces of equipment for the Core Workout. You can find the balls at most gyms now, and they can be purchased at sporting goods stores for around $25. (You also can consult www.coreperformance.com for ordering information.)

Physioballs come in various sizes. The rule of thumb is that the diameter (or height) of the ball should be 15 to 20 percent less than your inseam. The ball should be firm, not squishy.

The object of physioball exercises is to challenge your normal range of motion and in the process improve your balance, coordination, and stabilizing strength. But those are only a fraction of the benefits. Physioball movements are ideal for building pillar strength, since they increase *proprioceptive* demand (which we discussed in the Movement Prep chapter), while focusing on shoulder, hip, and core stability. And even that benefit doesn't do justice to the Physioball Routine. It's also fun. You may find it's the part of the Core Workout you most look forward to.

Let's look more closely at proprioception, the body's instant-messaging system: The unstable surface of the physioball forces your

CHOOSING THE RIGHT SIZE ■

YOUR HEIGHT	BALL HEIGHT	BALL SIZE
Up to 4 ft. 10 in. (145 cm)	14 in. (35 cm)	Small
4 ft. 8 in. to 5 ft. 5 in. (140 to 165 cm)	18 in. (45 cm)	Medium
5 ft. 6 in. to 6 ft. 0 in. (165 to 185 cm)	22 in. (55 cm)	Large
6 ft. 0 in. to 6 ft. 5 in. (185 to 195 cm)	26 in. (65 cm)	Extra large
Over 6 ft. 5 in. (195 cm)	30 in. (75 cm)	Extra, extra large

CORE LIFE PRINCIPLE: PHYSIOBALL ROUTINE

Like the physioball, life is uneven, constantly changing, and unpredictable. The unstable surface of the physioball forces you to create stability within your body and mind by using the things you can control, such as the core or your feet, which are on the ground. From there you build stability through your hips, core, and shoulders. You don't know what life will bring any more than you know what to expect from the physioball. To prepare, understand who you are and what things serve as your cornerstones. They give you stability, enabling you to deal with challenges as they arise.

CORE LIFE ACTION: Is your life lacking balance in some area? Take a moment right now and jot down ways you can bring more balance to your life.

muscles to heighten their readiness and to call more muscles into action to help stabilize your body and control that unstable surface. The end result is that you've improved the strength and stability of your pillar—shoulders, hips, core—while getting those three areas to work better together. The exercises have also improved the activation and elongation of these muscles, much like Movement Prep exercises do, and produced better mobility and neurological control.

As an example, let's compare the basic pushup to the physioball version. If you do a set of pushups on the floor, you'll need some strength, but not a whole lot of balance, agility, or coordination. But what if I give you the added challenge of placing your hands on the ball? Now your body has to compensate to keep the ball from moving. Your central nervous system has to recruit more of your muscles, allowing you to remain balanced. More of those little

muscles in the shoulder are activated, creating more stability. When we're challenging the body's feedback system to make quick adjustments, we say the exercise is "proprioceptively enriched." (Impress your friends at the gym with *that* phrase.)

The Physioball Routine exercises are designed to help you develop this sense of proprioception, which is a key component of stability and is vital to everyday life. In the Movement Prep chapter, we used the example of slipping on ice and explained how those exercises helped your body brace itself for those no-notice moments. The proprioceptive improvements you'll make because of the Physioball Routine might help you avoid falling in the first place.

Another example is sports, especially contact sports. If you're knocked off balance playing soccer, football, or basketball, your body's awareness of where it is in space will be improved because of this heightened proprioception. As a result, you may land without turning an ankle or tearing a knee. Not only may you prevent injury, you also may be in a better position to react to what's happening in the game.

Don't worry if the routine seems awkward at first. Even gifted professional athletes have difficulty when they first use a physioball. But you'll find that you pick up the exercises quickly and experience an immediate benefit. People often tell me that they feel as if they've activated and stabilized muscles they didn't know they had.

There's also a great feeling of accomplishment for being able to perform on an unstable surface. You'll increase the degree of difficulty somewhat, but the benefit will increase exponentially, and you'll feel great knowing that you can do something many people cannot.

By now, most gyms should have at least one physioball in an appropriate size for you, if not several. If yours doesn't, ask that it buy one. Your club should be willing to spend $25 to bring its facilities into the 21st century. (Like most of the Core Workout, the Physioball Routine also can be performed comfortably at home.)

Don't be surprised if you're the only one doing physioball exercises in your gym. I know it can be uncomfortable to stand out, doing something that might strike some people as strange. Just remember that you're getting far more benefit from your exercises, using muscles others have not learned how to tap into. All that, and you're having fun, too.

SUMMARY: By requiring you to work on an unstable surface, the Physioball Routine helps improve hip, core, and shoulder strength and stability by challenging your sense of proprioception, forcing your body to use more muscles.

TIME CAPSULE: Once you've mastered the Physioball Routine, you can do an abbreviated version of the basic movements in just 5 minutes. If you're pressed for time, just doing the Physioball Routine is an excellent workout to challenge and improve your hip, core, and shoulder stability. Even if you don't have time for Movement Prep, the Physioball Routine is an excellent stand-alone workout.

A CD-ROM featuring video of these exercises is available at www.coreperformance.com.

KWAME HARRIS

NFL OFFENSIVE LINEMAN
DATE OF BIRTH: 3/15/82

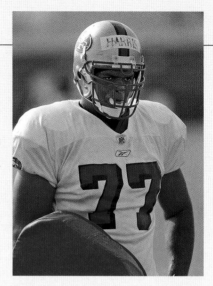

ON BALANCE AND THE PHYSIOBALL ROUTINE

When I was first presented with a physioball, I was skeptical. As a 6-foot-7, 310-pound football player, I was accustomed to pumping iron. How was this goofy contraption going to help me?

I quickly learned that the physioball could help me in areas that my high school and college training programs never addressed. I spent weeks doing shoulder-stabilization exercises, the same ones you'll soon learn, and the most remarkable thing was that when I went back to pumping iron, I was so much stronger because I had strengthened and stabilized all the little muscles that improve balance.

If you feel awkward or silly on the ball at first, don't worry. We all do. But you'll feel an immediate difference in how much more flexible your body is and the range of motion you have. You'll have control and awareness of muscles you didn't know existed.

I went to Mark Verstegen and his staff at Athletes' Performance to help improve my physical skills prior to the 2003 NFL draft, and they delivered big-time. I was able to better showcase my skills to prospective NFL employers. Along the way, I came to view the physioball as a metaphor for the importance of having balance in life. It's important not only to be open to new ideas and challenges but also to actively pursue varying interests that make you a complete person.

I'm a good football player, and the sport satisfies that primal, visceral part of myself like nothing else does. I'm passionate about playing football. But playing the piano or violin or reading a great book satisfies another part of myself, and that keeps me balanced.

During football season, I feel myself becoming testier, on edge, and while that helps on the field, it's important that I have other interests because I can't tie my entire personality to playing football or pursuing any other single endeavor. I need balance. There are times when I need to push the reset button because sometimes I can get too deep into one thing. Balance helps me take a step back.

Mark talks a lot about maintaining balance throughout your body and between opposing groups of muscles. You want to have good balance for muscle and joint stability and overall good health. You also want to have balance in life so that your interests and endeavors complement each other.

There will be times, of course, when you'll have to focus more on one area. But if you've achieved balance in your life, you'll find that you can raise your level of performance in everything that you do.

LATERAL ROLL

UNIT:
Physioball Routine.

OBJECTIVE:
To develop overall pillar strength (stability and strength in your shoulders, core, and hips).

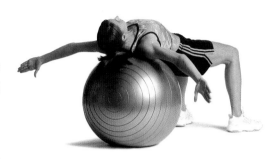

STARTING POSITION:
Lie supine (on your back) with the ball between your shoulder blades, hips fully extended, and knees bent to 90 degrees. Your arms are extended straight out to the sides. There should be a straight line from your knees to your shoulders and another straight line from hand to hand. Fire the glutes to keep your body in line. Keep your belly button drawn in.

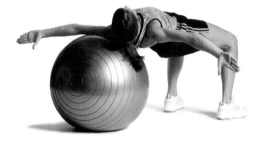

PROCEDURE:
Roll across the physioball, reaching as far to one side as possible, holding your arms parallel to the floor. Keep your hips tall.

COACHING KEY(S):
Keep your arms rotated so that your thumbs are back and down toward the floor, pulling your shoulder blades back and down.

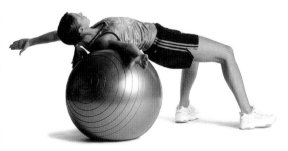

YOU SHOULD FEEL:
A stretch in your upper back and core and an activation of the glutes.

RUSSIAN TWIST

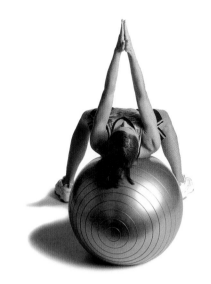

UNIT:
Physioball Routine.

OBJECTIVE:
To create increased mobility, stability, and strength between your shoulders and hips.

STARTING POSITION:
Lie supine on the ball, with your shoulder blades on the ball and hips tall.

PROCEDURE:
With shoulder blades back and down, extend your arms above your chest; your hands are either together or holding a weight plate. Keeping your hips tall, turn your shoulders to the right so that they're perpendicular to the ground while your hips stay horizontal. Twist back to the starting position and then to the other side.

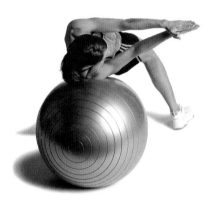

COACHING KEY(S):
When rotating to the side, be sure to fire (squeeze) the glute on that side to keep your hips flat.

YOU SHOULD FEEL:
A stretch in your core and an activation of the muscles of your hips and the sides of your waist.

PROGRESSION:
Hold a weight plate in your hands.

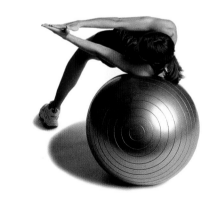

PLATE CRUNCH

UNIT:
Physioball Routine.

OBJECTIVE:
To develop overall core stability and strength.

STARTING POSITION:
Lie supine on the ball, arching your entire torso over the ball. Try to touch your shoulder blades, back, and glutes over the ball so that your abdominals are completely stretched. Hold the weight plate behind your head.

PROCEDURE:
Roll your hips and chest up at the same time while pulling your belly button in. Crunch from the top of your torso and then lower your hips and chest to the starting position.

COACHING KEY(S):
Arch your torso completely. Roll your chest and hips toward your belly button.

YOU SHOULD FEEL:
A stretch in your abs and core, followed by an activation of your midabdominal muscles.

PROGRESSION:
Hold the weight plate over your chest.

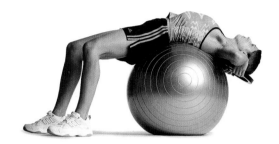
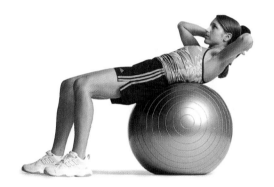
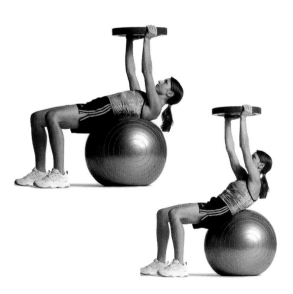

KNEE TUCK

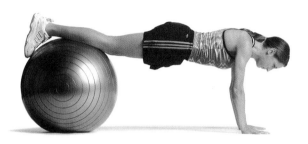

UNIT:
Physioball Routine.

OBJECTIVE:
To develop overall core and scapular stability. Also to stretch the muscles of your lower back.

STARTING POSITION:
Get in the pushup "plus" position (shoulder blades extended forward) with your shins on the ball.

PROCEDURE:
Pull your knees to chest until your toes are on top of the ball. Return to the starting position and repeat.

COACHING KEY(S):
Keep your belly button in and shoulders pushed away the whole time. Don't let your back sag.

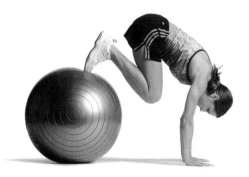

YOU SHOULD FEEL:
An activation in your core and shoulders and a stretch of your lower back.

PROGRESSION:

Use both legs bringing the ball in, just one taking it back out.

SECOND PROGRESSION:

Use one leg to bring the ball in and the same leg to take it out.

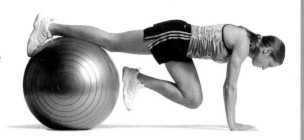

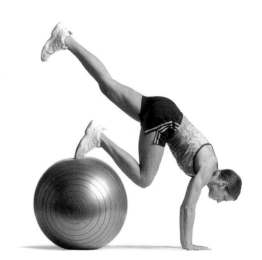

LYING OPPOSITES

UNIT:
Physioball Routine.

OBJECTIVE:
To develop posterior (back) stability and strength. Also to work the cross pattern from your shoulder to the opposite glute, improving muscle-recruitment patterns.

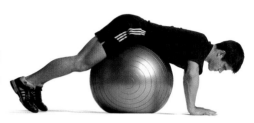

STARTING POSITION:
Lie prone (belly-down) on the ball, with your belly button over the center of the ball.

PROCEDURE:
Initiate the movement by activating the glutes. Elevate one straight leg toward the ceiling while extending your back and your opposite arm by using the scapula (shoulder blade) on that side. Go right leg/left arm, then left leg/right arm.

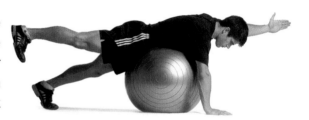

COACHING KEY(S):
Fire the glutes and move from the scapula so that the exercise benefits your entire back.

YOU SHOULD FEEL:
Contracting in your back, shoulders, and glutes.

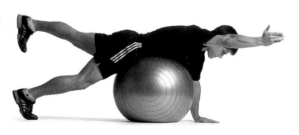

REVERSE HYPER

UNIT:
Physioball Routine.

OBJECTIVE:
To strengthen your lower back and glutes.

STARTING POSITION:
Lie prone (belly-down) on the ball, with your hands on the ground, feet on the ground, legs straight, and toes pointed up toward shins.

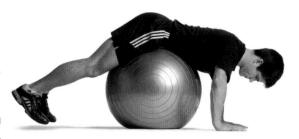

PROCEDURE:
Keeping your upper body still, activate the glutes to lift your legs up so that they're in a straight line with your upper body. You end up in a diagonal position, your face near the floor.

COACHING KEY(S):
Keep your shoulder blades back and down as you fire the glutes.

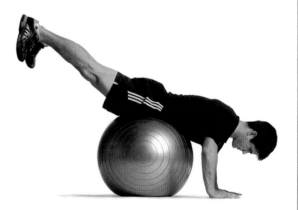

YOU SHOULD FEEL:
A stretch in the glutes and lower back, followed by an activation of those muscles.

PROGRESSION:
Drop one leg at a time, keeping the other in the air.

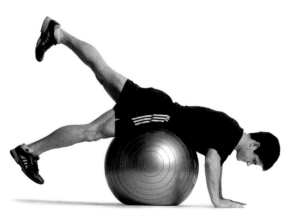

REVERSE CRUNCH

UNIT:
Physioball Routine.

OBJECTIVE:
To be able to rotate your pelvis and to keep your belly button drawn in.

STARTING POSITION:
Lie supine (with your back on the ground) and hook the ball between your heels and hamstrings.

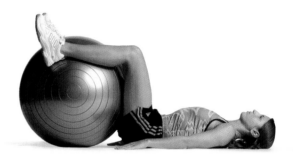

PROCEDURE:
Roll the ball up to your chest slowly, rolling your pelvis off the ground and tucking your knees to your chest.

COACHING KEY(S):
Keep your belly button in. Your abdominals must be drawn in to get the full benefit.

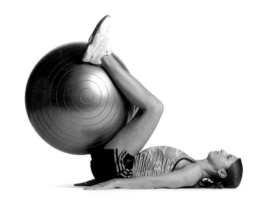

YOU SHOULD FEEL:
Activation of the core and stretch in your lower back.

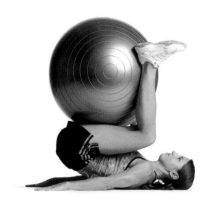

HIP CROSSOVER

UNIT:

Physioball Routine.

OBJECTIVE:

To build mobility and strength in your torso by disassociating your hips and shoulders.

STARTING POSITION:

Lie supine (back on the ground), with the ball between your knees and resting on the ground, your shoulders flat, and arms straight out to the sides. Tuck your heels toward your butt.

PROCEDURE:

Roll the ball over to one side until your knee touches the ground. Pull ball back and roll to the other side.

COACHING KEY(S):

Keep the ball on the ground throughout the movement.

YOU SHOULD FEEL:

A stretch in your core and torso rotators.

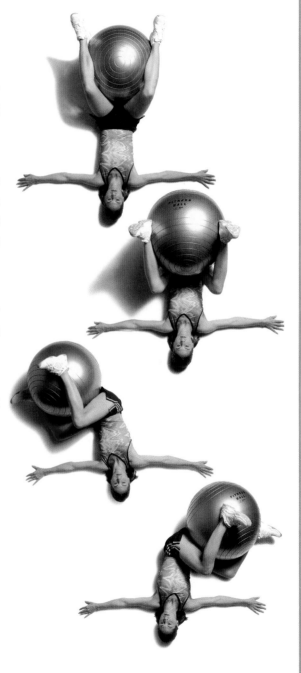

BRIDGING

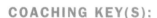

UNIT:
Physioball Routine.

OBJECTIVE:
To activate and strengthen the glutes and muscles of your lower back.

STARTING POSITION:
Lie supine on the ground, with your feet on the ball, toes pointed toward your shins, and shoulder blades pulled back and down.

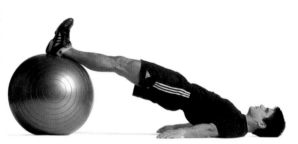

PROCEDURE:
Fire the glutes and raise your hips so that only your head, shoulders, and arms are touching the floor. There should be a straight line between your ankles and shoulders.

COACHING KEY(S):
Initiate the movement by firing the glutes and keep them fired at the top of the movement. *Note:* If you can't hold for the designated time, divide the time by 10 reps. (For example, 20 seconds becomes 10 reps of 2 seconds.)

YOU SHOULD FEEL:
Strengthening and activation of your hamstrings, glutes, and spinal erectors (lower-back muscles).

PROGRESSION:

Lift one leg for a 2-second hold, then switch legs.

SECOND PROGRESSION:

Lift one leg and tuck it to your chest.

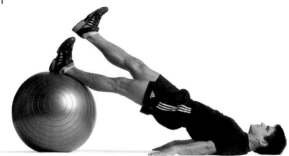

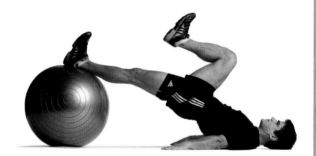

MIA HAMM

OLYMPIC AND WORLD-CHAMPION SOCCER PLAYER
DATE OF BIRTH: 3/17/72

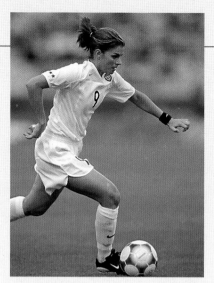

ON CORE PERFORMANCE *FOR WOMEN*

I was training at a track recently when I came across a heavyset woman walking along. I'm always inspired when I see such people working out, so I made it a point to talk to her.

She told me she was frustrated because she had been working out for 3 weeks and had yet to lose any weight. I told her not to be discouraged and suggested she find a way to measure her body's composition, the ratio of lean muscle mass to fat.

"I bet you've changed your body composition a lot," I told her. "If you measure your legs, hips, and waist, you'll see a huge difference. Not only that, but your muscles are a lot stronger."

I don't know if she followed my advice, but I do believe that too many people, especially women, become obsessed with the numbers they see on a scale. For the last two winters, I've trained with Mark Verstegen, and both times I've gone in hoping to lose some weight while getting stronger.

In both instances, I finished my 8-week program weighing pretty much the same—but I had transformed my body. I was so much stronger and had more lean body mass and less fat. Not only that, I also felt better from an endurance standpoint, ready to meet the challenges of professional soccer.

For me, Mark's *Core Performance* plan is directly applicable to what I do. If I still weighed what I did during my college career, I'd be broken in half. Top international players would push me off the ball. I'm 10 pounds heavier than I was in college, but none of it is fat. I've never felt faster and stronger than I have after working with Mark, who has taught me that a pound of fat takes up more space than a pound of muscle. So even though I weigh more than I did in college, I don't look bigger. In fact, I look leaner.

These days, women want to look athletic, and I think that's great. Look at athletes like sprinter Marion Jones or Brandi Chastain, my longtime teammate on the U.S. women's national team. They have incredible physiques. Who wouldn't want to look like that?

The great thing about this program is that it's all-encompassing. It covers strength, speed, flexibility, balance, and nutrition, along with the importance of rest and recovery. You're not just working one area, as you would in programs that just emphasize your butt or abdominal muscles. With Mark's program, you cover it all.

You'll work muscles you never knew you had. You'll spend a lot of time strengthening the smaller muscles around the hip, core, and shoulders, so you'll be able to support your joints, instead of putting strain on them when you bend over or lift something.

This program works areas that women seem to have trouble with, such as the thighs, stomach, and glutes, which is to say, your butt. Even when you're doing something like a dumbbell bench press, it's not just a strength exercise. You're using a technique that also works four or five other things, which help stabilize joints.

You'll not only feel stronger, you'll also be able to generate more force. Since starting Mark's program, I've noticed this when I shoot the ball. Even when I do a simple set of pushups, I feel that it's much easier to drive my body off the ground.

Don't worry if some of this seems strange or awkward at first. I've fallen off the physioball more times than I care to remember. Some of the best athletes in the world struggle with balance at times. Just remember that you're going to make progress, probably a lot faster than you might expect.

You don't have to be a competitive athlete to benefit from this program. Everyone needs to improve posture and pillar strength. My mom was a ballerina, and she was always telling me to keep my shoulders back, since I tended to have terrible posture. From working with Mark and strengthening all of the stabilizer muscles around the shoulder, I now keep my shoulders back naturally and have much better posture.

Another thing I love about Mark's program is that stretching is incorporated into the workout, beginning with the Movement Prep routine. By opening up the muscles throughout the workout, you get the full benefit of the exercise.

This is a program that men and women can do together. So many times I go into a gym and see some poor girl who is following her boyfriend's or husband's upper-body routine, trying to do five sets of a bench press with the heaviest weight possible. Meanwhile, the woman is saying, "I just want to get toned."

At Athletes' Performance, men and women work out together, performing many of the same movements and exercises. My husband, Nomar Garciaparra, and I do much of the same workout, though we each also do things specific to our sports.

Mark's great strength is his ability to take technical concepts and make them simple to understand. I know so much more about my body from working with him. Many people get frustrated with new workout routines because they either don't understand them or can't feel the results. With the Core Workout, you'll understand what you're doing, feel results quickly, and be eager to learn more.

I've often wanted to share this program with teammates but have shied away from it, since I don't pretend to be an expert on this. Now that Mark has written a book, I'm going to show it to teammates and friends. I'm excited that they can experience the same health benefits that I've enjoyed from working with him in person.

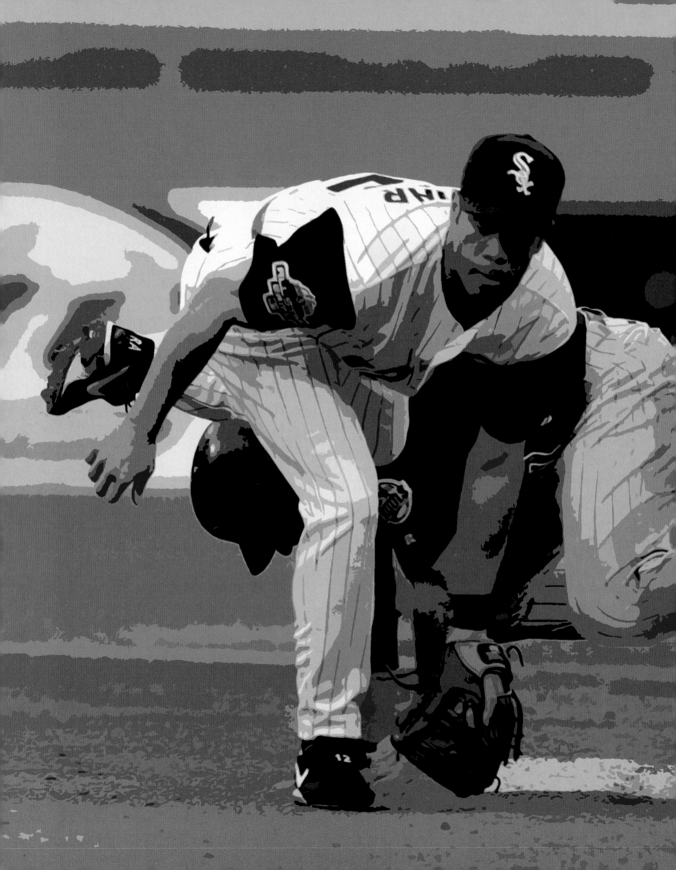

CHAPTER 8

ELASTICITY

T ake your left hand and place it on a flat surface, preferably a table. Raise your middle finger and push it down as hard as you can. Really slam that finger down.

Now relax your hand. Reach over with your right hand, pull that same finger back, and let it snap down. Go ahead. Do it! How much effort did it take to do that? Not much, but it generated so much more force than through the first method.

If you were to keep raising that middle finger on your own, you'd get tired. But if you can store and release that energy, lifting with your other hand, you can do it all day long and produce many times the power with a fraction of the effort.

This is a good illustration of elastic power. We want to be able to store and release energy efficiently. Everything we do has some sort of elastic component to it, whether it's walking, turning, going down steps, or playing sports. The more efficiently we can store and release energy, the less effort we have to give.

The golf swing is a great example of stored energy. You can't hit a golf ball very far if you run up to the tee and swing away. (*Happy Gilmore* to the contrary.) You generate torque and power as you go into the backswing, storing energy by stretching your hips, core, and shoulders. The better you do that, the more energy will be released to drive the ball down the fairway. Performing at any sport is a matter of effectively storing and releasing energy.

Think of your body as a pogo stick. The metal framework is analogous to your pillar, and the springs are like your muscles. We want our bodies to be able to store and release energy powerfully, just like that pogo stick.

Elasticity works in phases, starting with an elongation, in which the muscle puts on the brakes by lengthening and storing energy—as with golf's backswing. That's followed by a switch from the storing to the releasing of energy. It's important that we have excellent stability and proprioception during this period

CORE LIFE PRINCIPLE: ELASTICITY

Just as we store and release energy to become more elastic physically, we need to be pliable and elastic to overcome the speed bumps and barriers of life. Sometimes we have to give a little and bend to get past obstacles and grow. The more energy we can store and release from learning life's lessons each day, the easier it is to handle adversity and move forward. Elasticity also applies to giving and receiving. The more you give, the more you receive. Elevate yourself by helping others elevate themselves!

CORE LIFE ACTION: How can you help others to grow? Take a moment and list three people in your life and some concrete ways you can help them elevate themselves.

because we don't want to "leak" energy. From there, we release the energy and explode.

If we've stored and released energy correctly, we'll react like a Superball, which bounces very high. If energy is lost, we'll react more like a flat basketball, dropping on the ground with minimal bounce.

This unit will help immeasurably if you're looking to improve your vertical leap, but the benefits go beyond sports. Every move you make in life has an elastic component. When you walk, you stretch muscles. They release energy to propel you forward. Elasticity is your body's shocks and springs.

It's also a protective mechanism. If you slip and start to fall, your body needs to react quickly. A body with well-developed elasticity is going to contract the key muscles rapidly and make the corrections that keep you from tumbling.

Watch kids play, and you'll see how elastic they are. Of course, kids don't play as much as they used to, but when they do, you'll notice this. Kids run and jump on things. Kids' play is a developmental tool, not just mentally but also physically, in preparing their bodies for the demands of life.

Unfortunately, life deals us a double whammy when it comes to elasticity. Those of us who developed it as children lose it when we spend so much of our adult lives in front of computers and television sets. And the younger readers of this book may never have developed their full elastic potential, since kids today stop playing at earlier ages.

You may think you're compensating for all this with your exercise program, but if you train like most Americans, on jogging trails or in health clubs, you aren't. You may actually be making the problem worse.

Let's say you've spent some time in the weight room, and you have bigger muscles to

POWER AGING ■

Most adults know that muscles shrink with age—if you don't know, then you probably haven't passed 40 yet. Strength also deteriorates, which isn't exactly headline news. But most don't know that power—your ability to exert force at higher speeds—declines much faster than muscle mass or strength as you get closer to your senior-discount years.

And it's power, more than muscle size or strength, that determines whether you'll enjoy your golden years . . . or spend them in an assisted-care facility. The most obvious example is the sudden slip. An 80-year-old who's retained some of her physical power might catch herself before hitting the ground. An octogenarian without the ability to stop his fall might break a hip and spend the rest of his life as an invalid.

But none of us needs to suffer that fate. Power comes back fast when you focus on it in your workouts, as you will when you do the exercises in the Elasticity unit. Combined with the increases in strength, muscle size, flexibility, and function that you get from the other units in the Core Workout, the power you develop in this unit will make your body function as if it were years younger—maybe even decades younger, if you're over 50. And, even better, it just may save your life.

show for it. You'd think those muscles could generate power proportional to their size. They probably can't. There's not an exact correlation between the size of a muscle and its power. Bodybuilders, for example, have huge muscles, but their muscles aren't necessarily trained to generate a lot of power.

Now take someone like tennis player Meghann Shaughnessy, who is 6 feet tall and weighs 150 pounds. She produces as much power per pound as anyone because she has thoroughly developed her elasticity through training. Whereas traditional weight-room training emphasizes only slow, controlled ranges of motion, Meghann progresses toward elastic movement. She trains her body to store and release energy, to develop the

mechanism that makes the most efficient use of movement.

In this chapter, we're going to perform a series of jumps known as plyometrics. The jumping exercises—up and down, side to side, twisting back and forth—activate your body's central nervous system, stimulating the fast-twitch muscle fibers so that you can generate force as quickly and as efficiently as you need.

You'll also teach your body to *reduce* force more efficiently, which is just as important as generating it. A lot of injuries occur because you just can't decelerate quickly enough. Elasticity helps you slam on the brakes.

This chapter's exercises fall into three categories: short, long, and rapid response.

Rapid-response drills are low-force, high-speed, beginning activities to improve your ground reaction forces and your quickness.

Short-response activities help you hit the ground and immediately spring back off, improving your body's ability to be springy, or elastic. Think of a basketball being dribbled and the forces in motion, and you get the idea.

The long-response exercises use longer ranges of motion, and your feet will stay on the ground longer. But you'll produce higher levels of power with each repetition.

SUMMARY: You can improve your body's elasticity, its ability to generate and reduce force. By doing so, you'll make it more elastic and springy, much like a pogo stick. Elasticity decreases the potential for injury and allows you to produce more force (or less, if needed) in less time. Elasticity workouts are the perfect blend of stability, mobility, flexibility, strength, agility, and balance.

TIME CAPSULE: We're going to perform Elasticity exercises 2 to 4 days a week. They require no equipment, and in as little as 10 minutes they leave you feeling energized. For these exercises, it's important to maintain an "athletic position." Hold perfect posture, with shoulder blades back and down and tummy tight. Keep your legs slightly bent, with the hips sitting back and down, as if preparing to sit back in a chair. Your weight should be forward—on the middle to front of your feet, rather than on your heels. As you master this program and establish a base level of strength, you might find that when you're pressed for time, you focus on elasticity activities because they provide such a complete physical benefit.

A CD-ROM featuring video of these exercises is available at www.coreperformance.com.

ROBERTO ALOMAR

MAJOR LEAGUE BASEBALL PLAYER

DATE OF BIRTH: 2/5/68

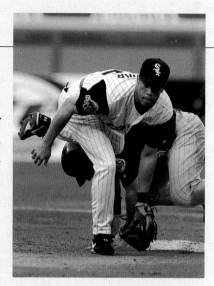

ON ELASTICITY AND BOUNCING BACK FROM ADVERSITY

I've been blessed with good elasticity. My body is naturally pretty springy, and that's helped me succeed as a baseball player, especially in the field as a second baseman. My ability to run, slide, lunge, and bounce back up has helped me win 10 Gold Gloves, awarded to the best fielders at their position in each league.

But as I've reached my midthirties, I realize that I no longer can get by on just natural ability. It's a good thing that I've been training with Mark for 7 years, because I've learned to train my body to bounce back from physical stress and to continue to meet the demands of playing baseball at the highest level. I actually feel as if I'm in better shape now than when I was 20, when I had no idea about conditioning, let alone a program like *Core Performance.*

In baseball, that elasticity helps me bounce back up after sliding to grab a ground ball. It helps me side-step a runner trying to knock me down at second base to break up a double play. It helps me get out of the way of a 95-mile-an-hour fastball coming toward my head at the plate.

This program has taught me that being elastic also applies to bouncing back from frustrations in life. In 2002, I had my worst season in baseball. It was my first season playing in New York, and I did not make a successful adjustment from playing in Cleveland. I also had a lot of nagging injuries. That season made me realize that I had to get in even better shape if I was going to continue to enjoy this great gift God gave me, the ability to play baseball.

The key is to try and maintain that elasticity, both mentally and physically. If you can do that, you're going to continue to be successful because you've already developed the wisdom that comes from experience. You just have to remain mentally and physically sharp.

This program as a whole will help you do that. But there's something about the Elasticity portion that makes you feel young. Maybe it's the jumping and bouncing and running. It makes you feel like you're a kid again, leaping and running without a care in the world.

My dad is 60 years old. He played in the major leagues, and he's kept himself in good shape. He often tells me he wishes that he had paid as much attention to his health as a player as he does now; he might have been able to play longer. I see how he's still able to move like a younger man, and it makes him seem like a younger person, both physically and mentally. He still moves like a professional athlete.

Look, we're all going to get old and face greater challenges and adversity. But there's no reason we can't keep our bodies—and our minds—as elastic and healthy as possible.

BASE ROTATION

UNIT:
Elasticity (rapid response).

OBJECTIVE:
Improves elasticity and creates disassociation between your shoulders and hips.

STARTING POSITION:
Stand with your shoulders square, your feet at a 45-degree angle.

PROCEDURE:
Rotate your hips to the right and left at a 45-degree angle. Shoulders stay stationary; use the hips only. Arms counterrotate, so when your hips are going left, your arms are going right.

COACHING KEY(S):
Imagine a large X on the floor. You're rotating your hips so your feet move to the ends of the X. Remember: Rotate from the core, not the shoulders.

YOU SHOULD FEEL IT:
In the core.

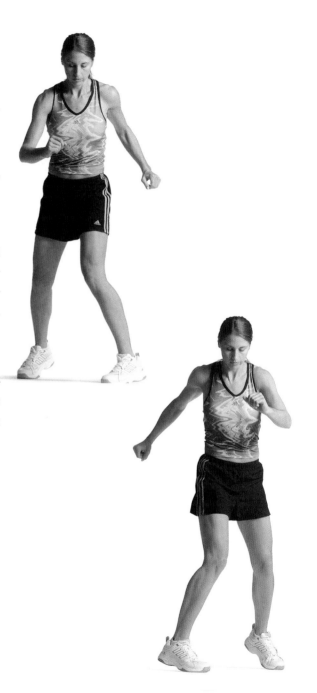

BASE SIDE-TO-SIDE

UNIT:
Elasticity (rapid response).

OBJECTIVE:
To create elasticity and quickness in your lower body with dynamic balance and stability.

STARTING POSITION:
Stand in an athletic position, with your feet outside your hips.

PROCEDURE:
Keeping both feet apart, jump 4 inches to the right, then 4 inches to the left, as if you were jumping back and forth over a line. Do this as rapidly as possible.

COACHING KEY(S):
As soon as you hit the ground, you should be springing back to the other side. This is not about height; it's about quickness in your lower body.

YOU SHOULD FEEL IT:
In the muscles around your hips, knees, and ankles.

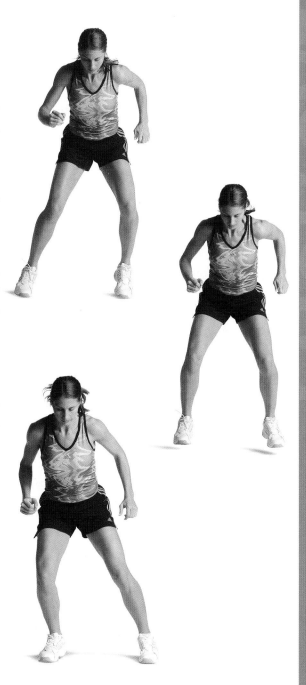

ONE LEG OVER THE LINE

UNIT:
Elasticity (rapid response).

OBJECTIVE:
To create quickness, elasticity, and dynamic stability in your lower body.

STARTING POSITION:
Standing with one foot parallel to a line, lift the opposite foot off the ground.

PROCEDURE:
Jump over the line and back as quickly as possible on one foot. This is a progression from the previous drill and requires more hip stability. Complete all the reps with one leg, then repeat with the opposite leg.

COACHING KEY(S):
Move as quickly as possible. Keep your hips stable underneath your pillar/torso.

YOU SHOULD FEEL IT:
In your quad, hip, and calf.

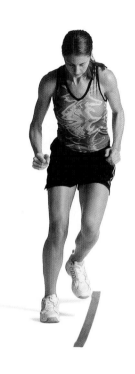

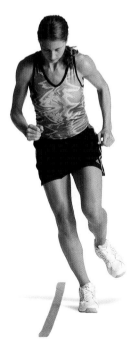

SPLIT JUMP

UNIT:
Elasticity (long response).

OBJECTIVE:
To improve balance, along with power and explosion in your hips and legs.

STARTING POSITION:
Take a large step forward, keeping your chest up, shoulder blades back and down, tummy tight, and knees and toes pointed straight.

PROCEDURE:
From the split-squat position, sit your hips back and down until your back knee nearly touches the ground. Hold this position for 2 seconds, then explode up, using your hips and legs and throwing your arms up at the same time. Extend your front leg and land back in the same split-squat position.

COACHING KEY(S):
Maintain good stability and balance upon landing.

YOU SHOULD FEEL IT:
In your hips and legs.

PROGRESSION:
Try alternate split jumps, switching your feet in the air with the back leg coming forward.

SECOND PROGRESSION:
Continue with alternate split jumps, but try to minimize the time on the ground.

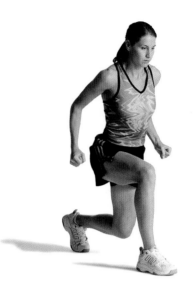
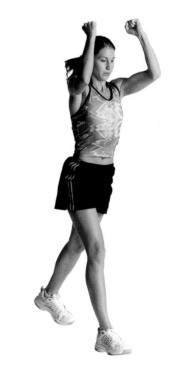

SQUAT JUMP

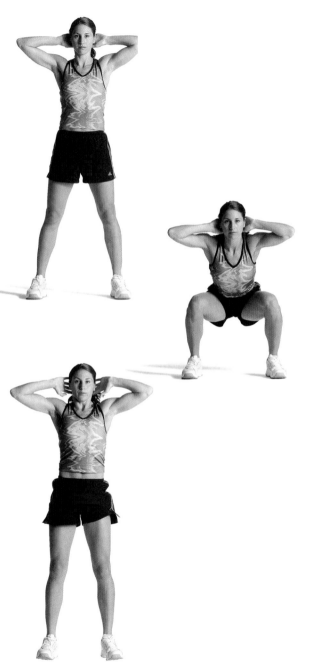

UNIT:
Elasticity (long response).

OBJECTIVE:
To build explosive power in your hips and legs.

STARTING POSITION:
Stand with perfect posture, with your feet outside your hips and your hands on your head.

PROCEDURE:
Sit your hips back and down until your thighs are parallel to the ground. Your back is erect, tummy tight. Jump, exploding from the glutes and quads. Extend your ankles, knees, and hips in a straight line and land in an athletic position.

COACHING KEY(S):
Extend your ankles, knees, and hips completely when jumping. Squeeze your glutes at the top of the movement and land with bent legs.

YOU SHOULD FEEL IT:
In your hips and legs.

WWW.COREPERFORMANCE.COM

PROGRESSION:

Move side to side, as shown.

SECOND PROGRESSION:

Move forward slightly with each jump.

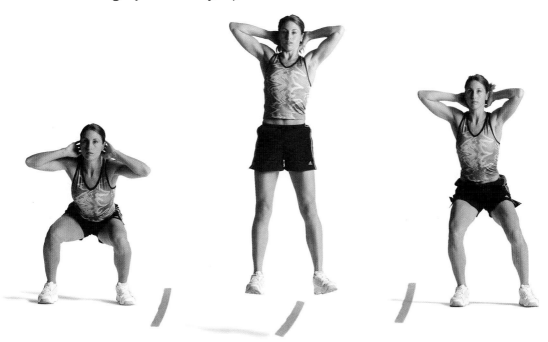

LATERAL BOUND

UNIT:
Elasticity (long response).

OBJECTIVE:
To build explosive lateral power in your legs.

STARTING POSITION:
Stand balanced on your right leg, with your left foot off the ground.

PROCEDURE:
Squat slightly with your right leg, then use your leg and glutes to jump laterally. Extend your ankle, knee, and hip and land on the opposite leg only, maintaining your balance. Repeat to the other side. Hold for a three count on each side.

COACHING KEY(S):
Explode out of your hips for maximum height. You're trying to jump as far laterally as possible for maximum height and distance. Land balanced; you should "stick it," as they say in gymnastics.

YOU SHOULD FEEL IT:
In your hips and legs.

PROGRESSION:
Move quickly on one side, holding on the other for 3 seconds.

SECOND PROGRESSION:
Move as fast as possible on both sides.

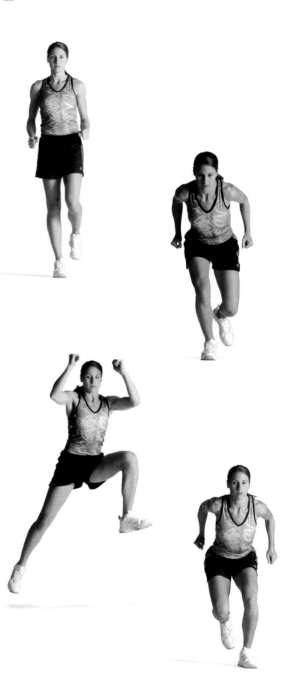

ANKLE JUMP

UNIT:
Elasticity (short response).

OBJECTIVE:
To build explosive power in your lower legs.

STARTING POSITION:
Stand with your legs straight, arms to the side, and toes cocked toward your shins.

PROCEDURE:
Bounce off the ground as quickly as possible by extending your ankles and pushing off the balls of your feet.

COACHING KEY(S):
Use the force of the ground to propel yourself up, landing on the balls of your feet. Keep legs unlocked. Pull toes back up after extending.

YOU SHOULD FEEL IT:
In your lower legs and feet.

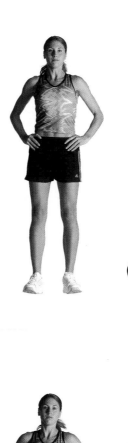
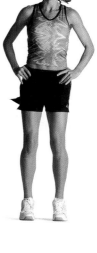
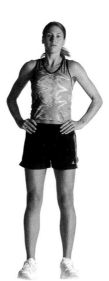

REACTIVE STEPUP

UNIT:
Elasticity (short response).

OBJECTIVE:
To improve explosiveness, stability, and balance in your lower body.

STARTING POSITION:
Place your right foot on a sturdy 6- to 10-inch box or step, with your arms cocked back.

PROCEDURE:
Jump vertically, driving off the top leg by extending your hip, knee, and ankle. Land in the same position, pause, and repeat. Finish all your reps with that leg, then repeat with the other.

COACHING KEY(S):
Throw your arms up but stop with your hands/fists at eye level. Land with your full foot on the box. Your torso should be leaning forward slightly upon landing, back leg bent slightly.

YOU SHOULD FEEL IT:
In your hips and legs. Overall, you should feel springy and powerful.

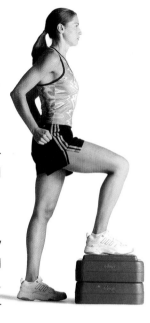

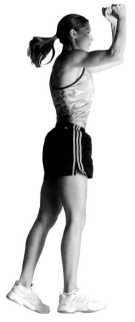

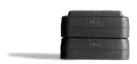

ELASTICITY

TUCK JUMP

UNIT:
Elasticity (short response).

OBJECTIVE:
To improve elasticity in your hips and legs.

STARTING POSITION:
Stand in an athletic stance.

PROCEDURE:
Jump off the floor, tucking your knees in front of your body up to waist height, then land back in an athletic stance.

COACHING KEY(S):
Synchronize your arm action with the jump. Be quick off the ground. Your knees should come up in front, progressing to waist height.

YOU SHOULD FEEL IT:
In your hips, legs, and calves.

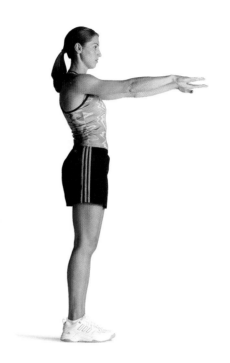

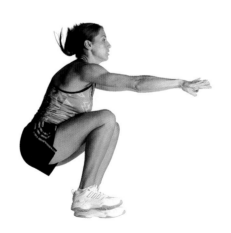

GET-UP

UNIT:
Elasticity (long response) to acceleration.

OBJECTIVE:
To build explosion and acceleration.

STARTING POSITION:
Assume and hold a pushup position, with your feet together.

PROCEDURE:
Explode forward into a sprint with piston-like leg and arm action. Run 10 yards.

COACHING KEY(S):
Hold perfect posture.

YOU SHOULD FEEL IT:
Everywhere. This is a total-body exercise.

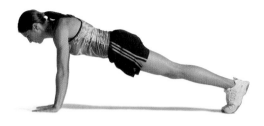

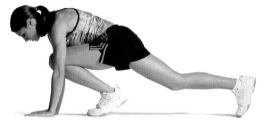

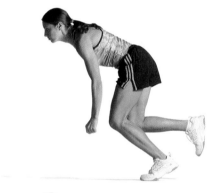

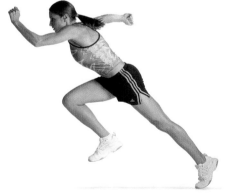

SIDE-TO-SIDE JUMP-TO-SPRINT

UNIT:
Elasticity (short response), lateral to linear movement.

OBJECTIVE:
To combine elasticity with acceleration.

STARTING POSITION:
From an athletic position, jump side to side over a line or an object no more than 6 inches high for the required number of reps. Upon landing the final rep, explode into a sprint for 10 yards.

COACHING KEY(S):
Hold perfect posture throughout. Accelerate with pistonlike leg action upon acceleration.

YOU SHOULD FEEL IT:
Everywhere, especially in your legs and hips.

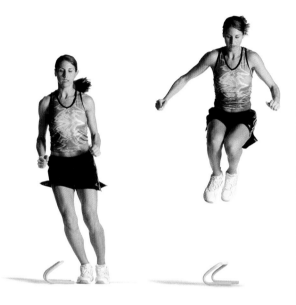

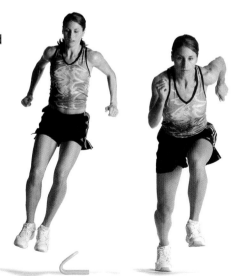

THREE-HURDLE DRILL

UNIT:

Elasticity (rapid response), lateral movement.

OBJECTIVE:

To improve quickness and your body's ability to perform cutting movements. Also to help your body benefit from ground reaction forces and improve coordination.

STARTING POSITION:

Lay three obstacles—towels, books, cups, or bricks, for example—each 2 to 3 feet apart from the other. Begin by straddling the first obstacle. Run laterally over the obstacles, never crossing feet. Rapidly reverse direction.

COACHING KEY(S):

Only your outside foot goes beyond the outside obstacles.

YOU SHOULD FEEL IT:

Everywhere. This is a total-body exercise.

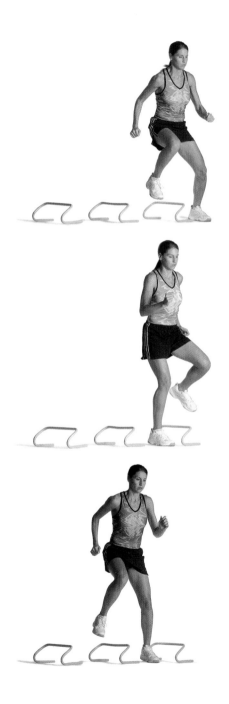

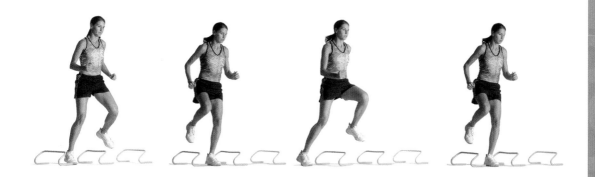

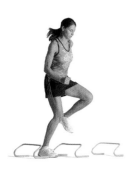

PLYO PUSHUP

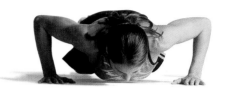

UNIT:
Elasticity/Strength.

OBJECTIVE:
To improve core stability and explosion of your upper body.

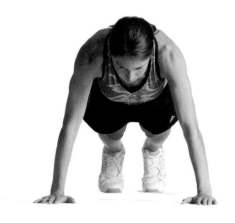

STARTING POSITION:
Get on all fours, with your tummy tight, pushing your chest away from the floor as far as possible.

PROCEDURE:
Lower your chest to the floor, then drive your body up explosively. Your shoulders and hands should be fully extended so your body is as far off the ground as possible. (If this is too difficult, you can rest your hands on a bench, as shown on opposite page, or against a wall.)

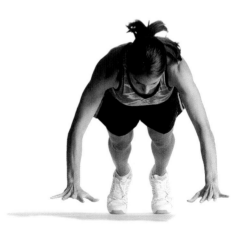

COACHING KEY(S):
Keep your body in a straight line. *Note:* The closer together your hands are, the more the exercise works your shoulders and arms.

YOU SHOULD FEEL IT:
In your chest, shoulders, and arms.

PROGRESSION:
Explode up into the air as high as possible.

SECOND PROGRESSION:
Add a clap while in the air.

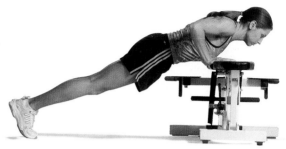

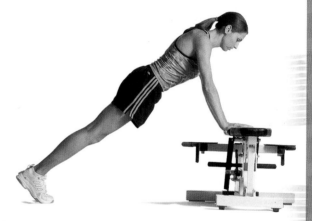

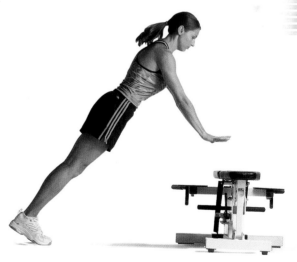

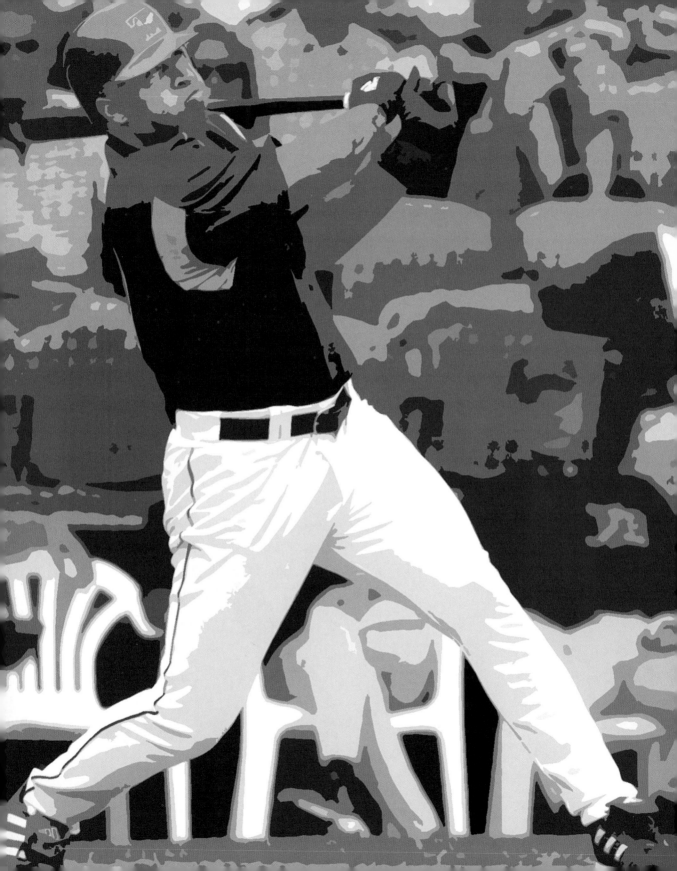

CHAPTER 9

STRENGTH

sn't it interesting that people rarely refer to *strength* training? Instead, they call it *weight* training or lifting weights. It's not just sloppy language. People have come to think of weights as a means to looking better—not to becoming stronger and more powerful or to improving balance and joint function.

But even if you accept that looking better is a perfectly fine goal on its own, you have to wonder why people go about it the way they do. To get better at something, even if it's just the appearance of your body, don't you have to make some sort of measurable progress? And yet, people rarely challenge themselves when they work with weights. They lift the same amount of weight for the same number of repetitions, year in and year out, never attempting to get stronger. Their bodies may make some changes at the start of their programs, perhaps even dramatic and noticeable changes. But then they stop challenging themselves to lift heavier weights, and their bodies stop changing. They may even backslide a bit, working out less often because of the boredom of a monotonous program.

You've probably figured out by now that,

with the Core Workout, boredom is never a problem. You'll always be challenged to improve. And in the Strength unit, you'll continually push yourself to get stronger.

But this part of the program is going to give you more than increased strength. You'll do exercises like the one-arm, one-leg dumbbell row, in which you'll do the familiar dumbbell-row exercise, but you'll do it standing on one leg. This way you'll recruit more muscles and improve their coordination. You'll certainly increase the strength of your back muscles and probably their size, but you'll also challenge your balance, flexibility, and joint stability.

Contrast that to the average muscle-building routines that you've done and that most of the people in your health club do. They look at their bodies as separate compartments, as in, "I'm going to train arms today."

CORE LIFE PRINCIPLE: STRENGTH

Strength is more than just physical power. Strength means staying the course, sticking to your beliefs, and not wavering from your goals and convictions. It takes strength to lead, to deviate from the norm, to resist peer pressure. It takes strength and character to motivate and empower people, instead of walking all over them to get where you want to go.

Think of strength as the accumulation of potential. You're building strength in this program to maximize your physical potential. Take that same approach to life, whether it's in your education, pursuit of knowledge, long-term financial investments, or the strong presence you project to those around you. The more strength you accumulate in all areas of your life, the more you will enjoy the benefits of that strength in the future. The greatest expression of strength is lifting others up.

CORE LIFE ACTION: What are your strengths? What are your weaknesses? Take a moment right now to make a list of each.

It's like having your Thanksgiving dinner spread out over 7 days, with turkey one day, cranberries the next, and pumpkin pie on the final day of the week. The joy of the Thanksgiving meal is in the total feast, not the individual dishes.

With the Strength unit of the Core Workout, every workout is a banquet.

The Strength chapter of the Core Workout includes some familiar exercises, like the bench press and the dumbbell bench press. But forget about doing the familiar three sets of 10. We're going to vary the number of sets and repetitions constantly and change the order of the exercises, too. I'll also give you the option of varying the tempo—the pace with which you raise and lower the weight—depending on what physical response you're looking to achieve.

We make these changes to challenge your body, systematically and constantly. Those challenges have a number of positive effects. Some are obvious: improved strength, more muscle, less fat. Some are psychological: You'll notice that strength training is fun again, just as it was when you first started. Or, if you've never thought moving iron was fun, you'll notice that this strength program is more enjoyable than any you've tried. When you get tired of iron, and its limitations, hopefully you'll be able to experience the true high performance of Keiser pneumatic equipment, which lets our athletes to train at any amount of resistance, in any plane, and at any speed, allowing us unlimited performance improvements.

Other effects are more subtle. For example, systematic changes in your routine prevent your body from reaching a plateau. If you've never reached a plateau before, you probably won't notice that you aren't on one. The constant variety also targets the muscle groups that complement and assist the ones you care most about. When you strengthen these traditionally neglected muscle groups, you make progressive improvements that you wouldn't make if you were doing the same thing week in and week out.

Along with all that, we're going to make the most efficient use of the time spent in the weight room. Too many people do a set and then sit around chatting for a few minutes before doing another. It's important to recover between sets, but in this program you'll recover without wasting time. And in the process, you'll get better results.

The key is supersets—a set of one exercise, followed by a set of a different exercise that involves an opposite movement. So if we do a pushing exercise, such as a bench press, we might follow it with a pulling exercise, such as a dumbbell row. When one set of muscles is working, the opposite set of muscles is resting. Not only is this a time-efficient way to train, it also produces better performance in the actual exercises, since the process allows the non-working muscles to recover faster while their opposing muscles work.

We're also going to combine exercises to form complexes. So rather than doing an exercise and then stopping to recover, we'll follow the first exercise with a similar movement to maximize the just-worked muscles' power.

Here's an example: You do a set of split squats (also known as a stationary lunge), then immediately do a set of split jumps. The second movement is similar to the split squat (you may remember it from the Elasticity unit), but instead of holding a barbell across your shoulders or dumbbells in your hands, you use your body weight and force your muscles to generate power after they're excited from generating strength.

Thus, we bring an elastic element to strength training. If we're going to take the time to develop strength and excite the nervous system through split squats, why not make the most of it by doing something that uses the same muscle-recruitment patterns and then apply it with much greater speed to get the nervous system and elastic properties involved?

It's all part of that banquet we talked about earlier. We want to be able to increase the range of motion with Movement Prep, then develop force through a strength exercise, and then contract powerfully through that new range of motion to enhance elastic properties.

All of which is a big departure from traditional, bodybuilding-based workouts. Bodybuilders aren't rewarded for being explosive and elastic, or to have greater flexibility or joint stability. They also, traditionally, do their exercises in one plane of motion. Many divide their workouts so they do "pushing" and "pulling" movements on separate days, but never advance beyond those single-plane exercises. In the Core Workout, we're going to include exercises that challenge you to move within all three planes of motion. The lifting and chopping movements, for example, will force you to rotate, something bodybuilders almost never do unless they're working their abs or cheating to lift heavier weights on one-arm rows.

Traditional weight-lifting programs take the right approach in having you do two or three sets of 10 reps initially. But that's just a starting point in the Core Workout. We're going to increase the quality and intensity of the exercises you do, and the way you do them, throughout the program. You'll build strength and muscle mass while increasing flexibility, balance, and elasticity, rather than diminishing those qualities as you get bigger and stronger.

SUMMARY: Traditional, bodybuilding-based strength-training programs focus on one-dimensional movement and working body parts. The Core Workout trains body *movements* so you increase levels of strength, lean body mass, stability, and mobility.

TIME CAPSULE: We'll perform the strength unit one to four times a week, 10 to 60 minutes a day. To make the most efficient use of our time, we will perform supersets and complexes to get more quality work done.

A CD-ROM featuring video of these exercises is available at www.coreperformance.com.

VERNON WELLS

MAJOR LEAGUE BASEBALL PLAYER
DATE OF BIRTH: 12/8/78

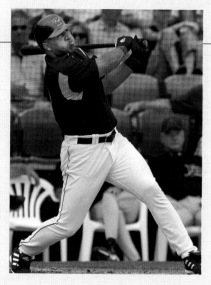

ON STRENGTH, CHARACTER, AND CONVICTION

By now, you've realized that strength comes from inside. It starts from the core, whether it's your physical strength or the core beliefs that give you a strong foundation for success. Working with Mark, I've come to understand the importance of including exercises that work the smaller muscles that provide support and stability in my hips, shoulders, and core. Strength isn't a matter of becoming huge but rather developing that pound-for-pound power that can make a wiry guy or petite woman every bit as strong as someone much larger.

Core Performance has helped me develop mental strength as much as my physical power. It's been said that 80 percent of baseball is mental. That also applies to golf and other sports, and even to life itself. If you have mental strength, that strength of character and of your convictions, then you'll be able to weather bad periods and stay strong no matter what happens. Having physical strength on top of that makes you even more of a powerhouse.

At Athletes' Performance, Mark emphasizes the connection between this pillar strength and the strength of our core beliefs. For me, I draw great strength from my family and religious faith. I have a beautiful wife and a young son, and church plays a prominent role in my life. They all make me strong enough to play baseball at the highest level and to get through life with peace and happiness no matter what happens. When you have those core beliefs, life is so much easier.

Don't get me wrong; I understand how fortunate I am to play baseball for a living. Compared to most people, I have few worries. But I know that when challenges and obstacles come up in my life, as they inevitably will, I'll be prepared to face them because of the strength of my beliefs as well as the pillar strength I've built through this program. And they do go hand in hand. It's possible to go through this program from purely a physical standpoint and experience tremendous results. But you'll get even more out of it if you try to define and strengthen your core beliefs along the way.

I've never thought of myself as a leader in the traditional sense, although I have been the team representative of the Toronto Blue Jays since I was 23. I kind of got drafted into the situation; no one else, it seemed, wanted to do it. Yet the role seems to fit. It's easy for people to come and talk to me no matter what I'm going through. I tend to walk with my head up—with perfect posture, as Mark might say—and that rubs off on other people.

My big-league baseball career is only a few years old. I have a lot of work to do. But with pillar strength and core beliefs, I have built a strong foundation to pursue my dreams.

ALTERNATE DUMBBELL BENCH PRESS

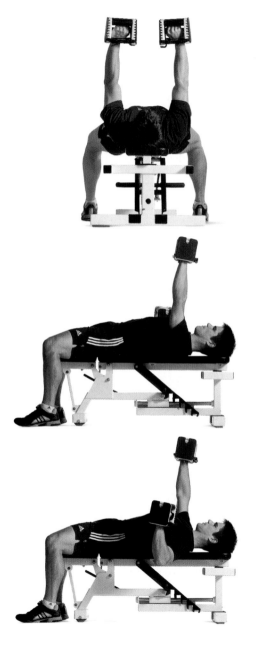

UNIT:
Strength.

OBJECTIVE:
To improve the strength of your chest, shoulders, and triceps while stabilizing your shoulders.

STARTING POSITION:
Lie supine (faceup) on a bench, holding dumbbells at the outside edges of your shoulders, palms facing your thighs.

PROCEDURE:
Lift both dumbbells straight up over your chest. Keeping one arm straight, lower the other dumbbell, touch the outside of your shoulder, then push it back up. At the top of the movement, "plus" (push farther) with both hands, as if trying to punch the ceiling. Then repeat with the other arm.

COACHING KEY(S):
Make sure to stabilize your extended arm and take the active dumbbell through a full range of motion. "Plus" at the top with both hands.

YOU SHOULD FEEL IT:
In your chest, shoulders, and triceps.

STRENGTH

BENCH PRESS

UNIT:
Strength.

OBJECTIVE:
To improve strength and power in your chest, shoulders, and triceps.

STARTING POSITION:
Lie supine on the bench, with your feet on the floor. Your shoulders and hips remain in contact with the bench the entire time. Grasp the bar (or hold the dumbbells) just wider than shoulder width, and hold it with straight arms over your shoulders.

PROCEDURE:
Breathe in, lowering the bar to the lower part of your chest. Drive the bar forcefully back to starting position. Extend your arms and shoulders fully at the end of each repetition.

COACHING KEY(S):
Keep your feet on the floor and your hips and shoulders on the bench at all times. Keep your head straight.

YOU SHOULD FEEL IT:
In your chest, shoulders, and arms.

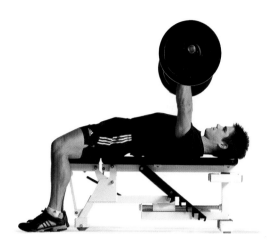

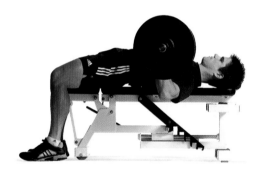

ONE-ARM, ONE-LEG DUMBBELL ROW

UNIT:
Strength.

OBJECTIVE:
To develop upper-back strength and power, along with hip stability. Also to work the cross-body connection from your shoulder to the opposite glute.

STARTING POSITION:
Stand on one leg, grasping a stable surface in front of you (such as a dumbbell rack) with one hand.

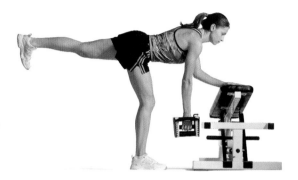

PROCEDURE:
Bend by dropping your chest and lifting the leg opposite your free hand to create a perfect *T* with your body. Grab a dumbbell with your free hand. Pull it to the side of your waist and then lower it. Perform the designated number of reps with one arm, then repeat with the opposite arm and leg.

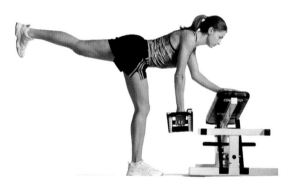

COACHING KEY(S):
Move your shoulder, not your arm, to initiate the row. Keep your back level—your shoulders should stay parallel to the floor—and fire the glute of your extended leg to keep it parallel to the floor. Extend the leg opposite the hand doing the lifting.

YOU SHOULD FEEL IT:
In your back, lat, and shoulder.

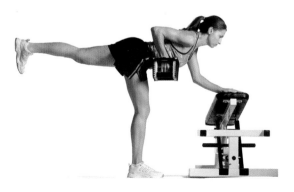

DUMBBELL FRONT SQUAT-TO-PRESS

UNIT:
Strength.

OBJECTIVE:
Total-body strength and power.

STARTING POSITION:
Stand holding dumbbells at shoulder height, with your elbows resting on your ribs, palms facing each other.

PROCEDURE:
Initiate the movement with your hips, squatting back and down until the tops of your thighs are parallel to the floor. Explode out of your hips and quads, using that momentum to drive the weights off your shoulders and overhead. You should finish with straight legs and arms. Lower the dumbbells back to your shoulders, then drop back into a full squat and repeat.

COACHING KEY(S):
Keep your weight on your heels when squatting—never let your weight go forward onto your toes.

YOU SHOULD FEEL IT:
Pretty much everywhere. This is a total-body exercise.

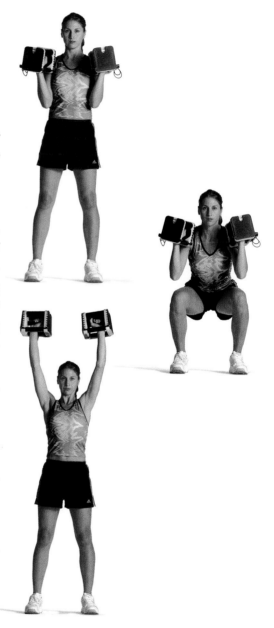

SPLIT SQUAT/LUNGE

UNIT:
Strength.

OBJECTIVE:
To increase balance and strength in your hip and leg muscles.

STARTING POSITION:
Set a bar across your shoulders or hold dumbbells at arm's length at your sides. Step out into a lunge.

PROCEDURE:
Lower your hips toward the floor by squatting back and down. Without letting your back knee touch the ground, return to the starting position by driving your weight back up with your front leg. Do all the reps with that leg forward, then switch legs and repeat.

COACHING KEY(S):
Don't let your front knee slide forward over your toes; if it does, start over again with your front foot farther forward.

YOU SHOULD FEEL IT:
In your hips and the front of your legs.

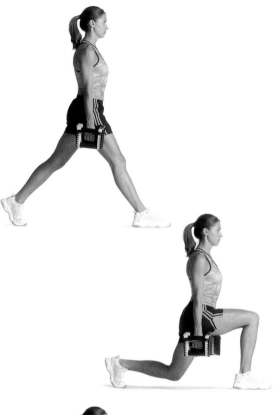

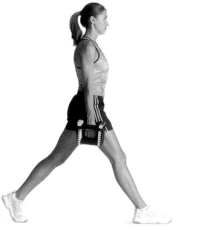

STRENGTH

PROGRESSION:

Place your back foot on a box or bench (this move is also called a Bulgarian split squat).

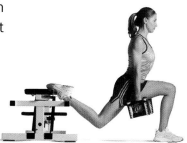

SECOND PROGRESSION:

Step forward on each repetition, alternating legs as you go (these are walking lunges).

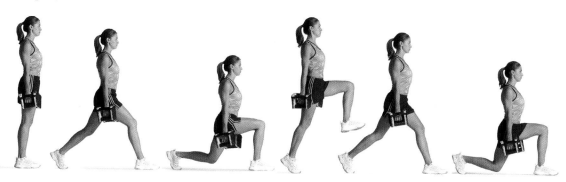

THIRD PROGRESSION:

Place your back foot on a slippery surface, such as a wood or linoleum floor. Or put a magazine or file folder on the carpet and place your foot on that.

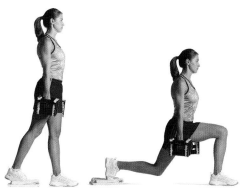

FLOOR/PHYSIOBALL LEG CURL

UNIT:
Strength.

OBJECTIVE:
To improve strength and stability in your glutes, hamstrings, and lower back.

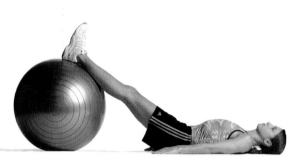

STARTING POSITION:
Lie supine (faceup) on the floor, put your heels on the ball, pull your toes up toward your shins, and pull your shoulder blades back and down.

PROCEDURE:
Squeeze your glutes until your body is in a straight line from ankle to shoulder. Keeping your hips tall, pull your heels in toward your glutes. Let the ball roll back slowly as you straighten your legs, keeping your hips elevated. Stay in the bridge for all your repetitions.

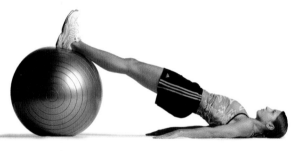

COACHING KEY(S):
Be sure your glutes stay activated the entire time. Don't let your hips drop as you pull your heels in. *Note:* If you don't have access to a physioball, you can do this exercise on a smooth floor (wood or linoleum). Put a towel beneath your heels to allow a smooth movement. Or, if you're using a carpeted floor, put a magazine or file folder beneath your heels.

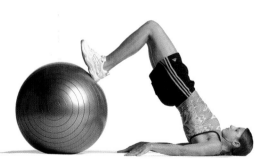

YOU SHOULD FEEL IT:

In your glutes, hamstrings, and calves.

PROGRESSION:

Use two legs to bring the ball in, one leg to let the ball out (not shown).

SECOND PROGRESSION:

Use one leg to bring the ball in, one leg to let the ball out. Tuck your other knee to your chest.

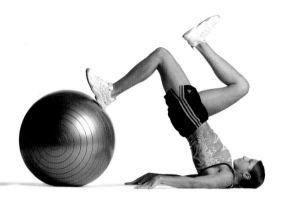

CABLE ONE-ARM ROTATIONAL ROW

UNIT:
Strength.

OBJECTIVE:
To improve stability and strength in your back, torso, shoulders, and arms.

STARTING POSITION:
Attach a handle to the low pulley. Kneel perpendicular to the cable machine, with your right knee and left foot on the floor.

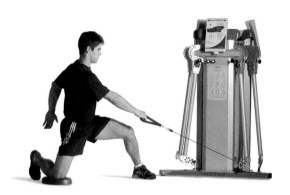

PROCEDURE:
Reach across your body with your right hand to grab the handle, turning your hips and shoulders to the machine. Now rotate your right shoulder back and pull the handle to your right hip (much like a dumbbell row). Do all your reps, then repeat with your opposite side.

COACHING KEY(S):
This movement should look and feel as if you're trying to start a lawn mower that doesn't want to crank. Don't forget to turn your shoulders and hips toward and then away from the machine with each repetition.

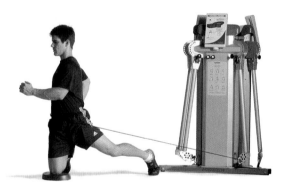

YOU SHOULD FEEL IT:
In the torso and hip rotators, waist, lats, arms, and rear shoulders.

STRENGTH

PROGRESSION:

Try these rows while seated on a physioball.

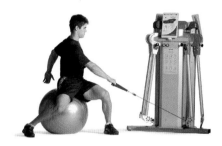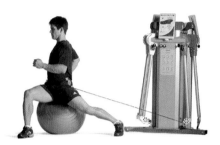

SECOND PROGRESSION:

Perform this exercise while standing.

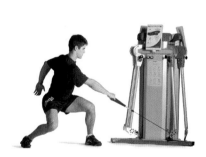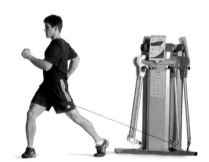

CABLE CHOPPING

UNIT:
Strength.

OBJECTIVE:
To improve stability and strength in your arms, upper back, and torso rotators; to improve rotational ability of your torso, upper back, and arms.

STARTING POSITION:
Attach a handle or rope to the high pulley. Sit on a physioball, perpendicular to the cable machine.

PROCEDURE:
Rotate your shoulders and grab the handle with both hands. Now pull the handle to your chest as you rotate away from the machine, continuing the momentum by pushing the rope down and away. Do all your reps, then repeat with your opposite side.

COACHING KEY(S):
Turn toward and away from the machine with each repetition. At the end of each rep, your chest should be up, your shoulder blades back and down, and your tummy tight.

YOU SHOULD FEEL IT:
In your shoulders, triceps, and abs.

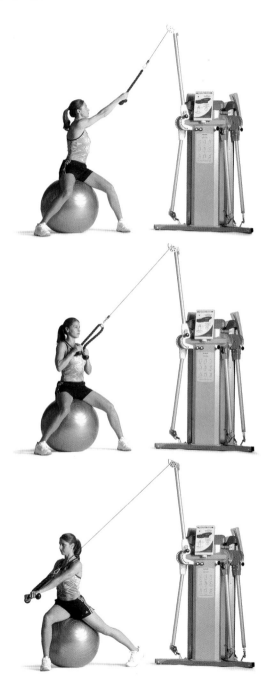

PROGRESSION:

Instead of using the physioball, start by kneeling on your outside leg, inside leg up, perpendicular to the machine.

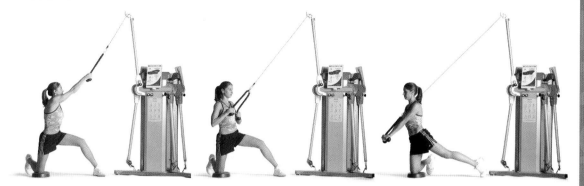

CABLE LIFTING

STRENGTH

UNIT:
Strength.

OBJECTIVE:
To improve your torso's rotational ability and to build strength in your upper back, shoulders, chest, and triceps.

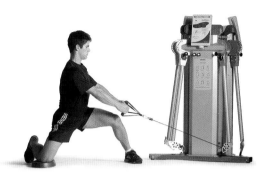

STARTING POSITION:
Attach a handle to the low pulley. Kneel on your outside leg, with your inside leg up, perpendicular to the machine.

PROCEDURE:
Grab the handle and turn your shoulders, keeping your chest up and tummy tight. Pull the handle up toward your chest while turning your shoulders and continue the motion by pushing it up and away. Lower your hands back toward your chest as you turn back to the machine. Do all your reps, then repeat with your opposite side.

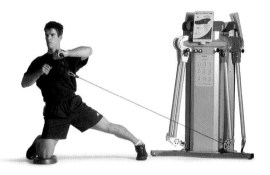

COACHING KEY(S):
Be sure to turn your shoulders. Your back should be turned to the machine at the end of the movement. Think of this as a combination of two familiar movements—upright row and incline press—but turned to the side and combined in one motion. Lower in the same pattern as you lifted.

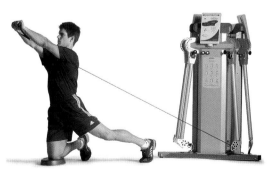

YOU SHOULD FEEL IT:
In your torso rotators, upper back, chest, and shoulders.

PROGRESSION:

Try this exercise while seated on a physioball.

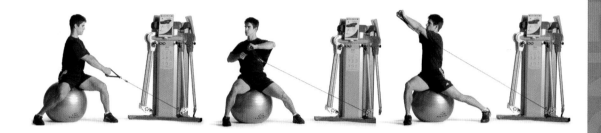

SECOND PROGRESSION:

Perform this exercise while standing.

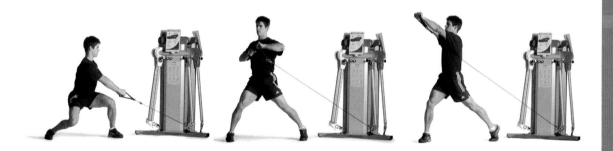

DUMBBELL PULLOVER EXTENSION

UNIT:
Strength.

OBJECTIVE:
To improve strength and coordination between the muscles of your upper back and triceps.

STARTING POSITION:
Lie supine on a bench, with dumbbells held with straight arms over your chest or eyes.

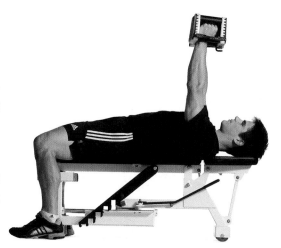

PROCEDURE:
Keeping your upper arms in the same position, lower the dumbbells until your elbows are bent 90 degrees. Now lower your upper arms until they're parallel to the floor. Now pull your arms back to the starting position, straightening your elbows on the way up. *Note:* If you have shoulder problems, just do the first half of the movement, bending your elbows and then straightening them.

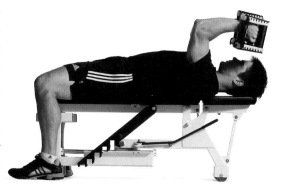

COACHING KEY(S):
Drop your hands first so that your elbows point up toward the ceiling, then drop your elbows.

YOU SHOULD FEEL IT:
In your upper back, lats, and triceps.

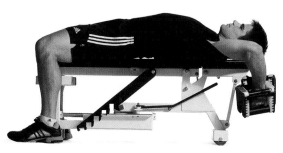

STRENGTH

SPLIT DUMBBELL CURL-TO-PRESS

UNIT:
Strength.

OBJECTIVE:
To build strength in your arms and shoulders, while stabilizing your hips and core.

STARTING POSITION:
Stand holding dumbbells at your sides. Rest your front foot on a bench or sturdy step at about midthigh height.

PROCEDURE:
Perform a biceps curl, rotating your palms so they're facing you. Then press the weight over your head, finishing with either the palms facing forward, in, or backward. Do all your reps, then put the opposite foot on the step for your next set.

COACHING KEY(S):
Maintain perfect posture, with belly button pulled in and shoulder blades pulled back and down.

YOU SHOULD FEEL IT:
In your biceps and shoulders and throughout your pillar.

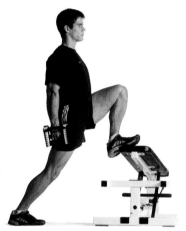

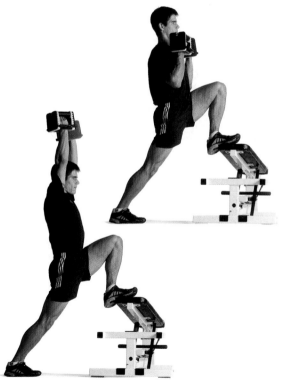

ROMANIAN DEADLIFT

UNIT:
Strength.

OBJECTIVE:
To build strength in your hamstrings, glutes, lower back, and upper back.

STARTING POSITION:
Grab a barbell with an overhand grip just wider than shoulder width, or stand holding a pair of dumbbells at your sides. Set your feet hip-width apart, with your legs in a fixed position but not locked at the knees. Your shoulders should be back and down and your weight on the back half of your feet.

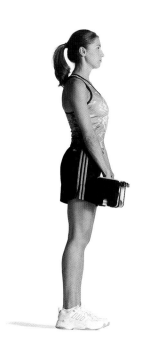

PROCEDURE:
Shift your hips back and lower the bar as far as you can while keeping your back straight. Fire your hamstrings and glutes as you return to an upright position.

COACHING KEY(S):
Your torso/pillar stays straight. Keep the bar or dumbbells close to your body, touching your legs or almost touching all the way up and down. Don't think of the exercise as bending forward; think of it as sitting back, but with your torso moving forward instead of staying upright. Keep your shoulder blades back and down throughout the movement.

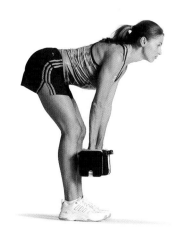

STRENGTH

YOU SHOULD FEEL IT:

In your glutes and hamstrings mostly, with some effort in your lower back and core. You may feel it in your upper back, since it's challenging to keep your shoulder blades retracted as the weight moves toward the floor.

PROGRESSION:

Try one-arm, one-leg dumbbell Romanian deadlifts.

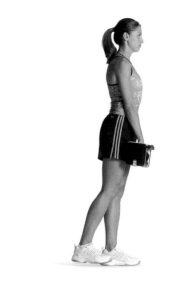

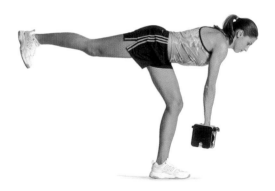

PULLUP

UNIT:
Strength.

OBJECTIVE:
To develop muscles of your upper back, shoulders, biceps, and forearms.

STARTING POSITION:
Grab a pullup bar with either an overhand or reverse (underhand) grip. (If you have access to a bar with handles, you can take a "neutral" grip, with palms facing each other.)

PROCEDURE:
Hanging from the bar, pull your shoulder blades back and down to lift your body up. Finish by pulling with your arms.

COACHING KEY(S):
Return to the fully extended position after each rep. If you can't do a pullup initially, perform a "horizontal" pullup by lying underneath the bar of a squat rack or Smith machine, as shown on next page.

YOU SHOULD FEEL IT:
Under and around your shoulder blades, backs of your shoulders, and your arms.

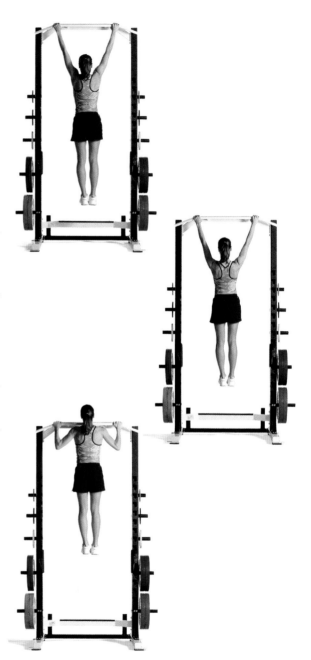

STRENGTH

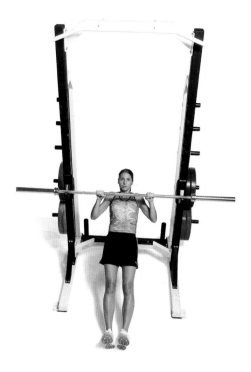

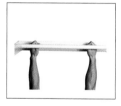

Neutral grip

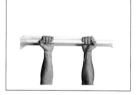

Underhand grip
(chinup)

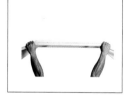

Wide overhand
grip (most difficult)

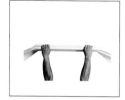

Normal
overhand grip

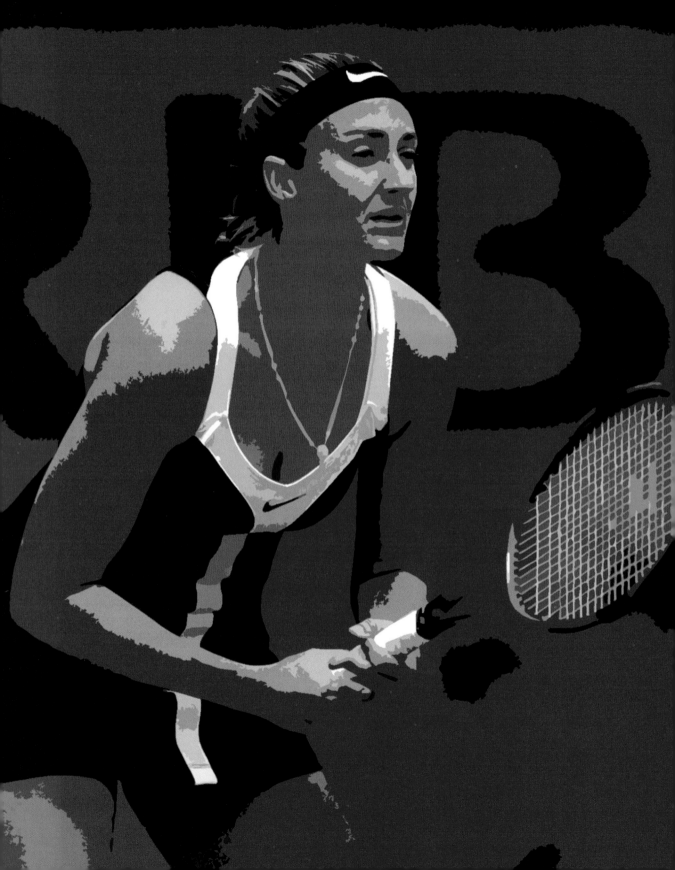

CHAPTER 10

ENERGY SYSTEM DEVELOPMENT

Everyone agrees that daily physical exercise is vital. The Surgeon General and the American College of Sports Medicine suggest that adults should engage in a minimum of 30 minutes of "moderately intense" physical activity every day.

But what constitutes moderately intense activity? Many exercise programs spell out the strength portion, then leave you to do cardio a few times a week. There are no specific instructions, and, as a result, most people just go for a leisurely jog. Others hop on a stationary bike for 30 minutes, reading the paper or watching CNN. Most people don't work nearly as hard as they should and thus waste time and fail to tap into their potential. They do the same thing every day, their bodies stop adapting, and they end up looking pretty much the same at the beginning and end of whatever program they're on.

I dislike the term *cardio* for that very reason. Over the years it's come to mean light exercise. At Athletes' Performance, we refer to cardio as energy system development, or ESD,

because we're not just burning calories for the sake of burning them. We're also improving the function of the heart and lungs and building endurance. In short, we're teaching the body to tap into new energy levels.

There's an element of ESD in the entire Core Workout. If you're moving quickly through all of the routines, you're going to achieve a phenomenal ESD result. Don't feel bad if you don't have time for ESD, because even without it you've had a great workout. If you have the time, you can achieve an even greater impact on your health, body composition, and performance level by performing the ESD unit.

Most fitness programs—no matter their goals—fall short of challenging your body, especially when it comes to energy system development. For most people, "running" is

CORE LIFE PRINCIPLE: ENERGY SYSTEM DEVELOPMENT

Just as you learn to tap into new energy levels to enable your body to work at higher capacities, recognize that you can use this same process to meet the challenges of life. If you can focus and work extremely hard for short bursts, you'll be so much more productive, especially if you've developed your energy levels to the point where your lowest "zone" is much higher than that of the average person. The better we can stay focused and productive at a high level, the more quickly we'll be able to drop back down and enjoy everything else life has to offer.

CORE LIFE ACTION: What areas in your life require more energy, a higher level of performance? Jot down a few of those areas now.

synonymous with "jogging." If you tell someone you run, they automatically ask, "How far do you run?" No one ever asks, "How fast do you run?"

Distance running puts a tremendous amount of stress on the body. Each time the foot hits the ground, the force is equivalent to as much as seven times your body weight. The cumulative trauma can be devastating, especially if you have poor running mechanics. It's like driving a car that's slightly out of alignment for a few thousand miles. Eventually, it's going to break down.

When you were a kid, it never occurred to you to try to run a long distance. To you, "running" meant getting somewhere, and getting there fast. You also probably realized that fast running was the ultimate expression of power and athleticism. The best baseball, football, and basketball players in your school or peer group were probably also the fastest. And they weren't weaklings either. The guy who got chosen first in street football or schoolyard dodgeball was probably not only the fastest but also the most powerful, the guy who could throw hardest and hit or kick a ball farthest.

And yet, we somehow forget all that as adults. We never equate the qualities we want—bigger muscles, a leaner body—with speed and explosive power. It's not too late. When you get faster, you improve your muscle size and power, the efficiency of your nervous system, and even your flexibility.

All that, and you burn calories, too. Have you ever seen a fat sprinter?

Before I explain how I want you to get these benefits, I want you to forget everything you currently believe about cardio work. Forget keeping your heart rate in some "fat-burning" zone. Forget plodding along with the vague goal of increasing the distance you can plod. Instead of training like a plow horse, you're going to train like a thoroughbred.

No, I'm not going to make you head to the track and train like a middle-distance runner, although you're welcome to do your ESD work there if you like. For convenience, you'll probably want to work on a stationary bike, stairclimber, or treadmill at the gym. Even better is to find a hill or stairwell somewhere nearby. If you're city-bound, parking garages are perfect for uphill running. Sprint up the ramps and walk down.

Specifically, I want you to develop three different energy systems. First, you're going to develop and improve your body's *lactate threshold,* its capacity to do high-intensity work for up to 3 minutes. The ESD unit of the Core Workout is a form of interval training in which you will alternate periods of intense exercise with less strenuous periods.

You'll also work on your *alactate power,* your body's ability to do high-level work for periods of up to 12 seconds. The exercises of the Elasticity unit are good examples.

Finally, ESD will help build your *aerobic* system, the ability to work beyond 3 minutes and help you recover from your bouts with the lactate threshold. For instance, if you're sprinting up hills and walking down, you're using the lactate system on the way up and the aerobic system on the way down. In this case, the aerobic system enhances your recovery from these intense bursts of energy.

You'll only work at the same effort level for an extended period of time, as you would with traditional cardio exercise on regeneration or recovery days. Instead, you're going to take the same period of time and develop the ability to perform at a more intense level. You're improving your energy levels, gaining physical strength and stamina without investing additional time.

You'll work within three heart-rate "zones." To calculate your maximum heart rate, begin by subtracting your age from 220. If you're 40 years old, your maximum heart rate is 180. (It may actually be higher or lower than that, but this is close enough to allow productive workouts.) Multiply that rate by 60 and 70 percent to determine zone 1. Multiply it by 71 and 80 to determine zone 2, and multiply by 81 and 90 percent to determine zone 3.

These are general guidelines. You may need to raise or lower the numbers by 10 beats across the board. If nothing else, you will need to raise them as your ESD improves.

If you're 40 years old, your starting numbers will read as follows:

- Zone 1 = 108 to 126
- Zone 2 = 127 to 144
- Zone 3 = 145 to 162

ESD work will involve periods of intense work followed by slightly easier work. You could sprint up a hill and walk down. Or pedal as hard as you can on a bike for a period, then return

ESD WORKOUTS ■

WORKOUT #	TOTAL TIME	WARMUP	SETS
1 Aerobic/Recovery	12 min.	n/a	1
2 Aerobic/Recovery	20 min.	n/a	1
3 Aerobic/Recovery	30+ min.	n/a	1
4 Lactate Capacity	15 min.	3 min./Z1	1
5 Lactate Capacity	15 min.	3 min./Z1	1
6 Lactate Capacity	17 min.	3 min./Z1	1
7 Lactate Capacity	19 min.	3 min./Z1	1
8 Lactate Power	15 min.	3 min./Z1	2
9 Lactate Power	15 min.	3 min./Z1	1
10 Lactate Capacity	11 min.	3 min./Z1	1
11 Lactate Power and Capacity	15 min.	3 min./Z1	1

to a slower pace. Spinning classes, for example, provide good ESD work.

In the early stages of the Core Workout, you'll work mostly in the first two zones. Gradually, you'll work your way into zone 3. The ESD portion of your workout will vary between 12 and 30 minutes. Since you'll also be doing some combination of other units, it might be convenient to do ESD work on a treadmill, stationary bike, or other machine in the gym. Many of these machines are equipped with heart-rate monitors. You grasp the handles, and within seconds the machine gives you a reading. (Some even tell how many calories you've burned, though this is accurate only if they calculate the calories based on your weight.)

You're probably thinking that 12 to 30 minutes on a machine will be easy, right? Not in the Core Workout. If you have a 2-minute zone 2 interval, you have to work as hard as possible on that piece of equipment to maintain your heart rate in that zone. (Be sure to set the machine on manual so that you control the pace, and don't cheat yourself by leaning on the equipment.)

With most cardio work, people believe that they're exercising much harder than they really are. Some gyms have "perceived exertion charts" on the wall where people can attach a number figure to how they feel. Most people go by sweat, which often is a function of how long they've been on the machine (if not the temperature in the room), and not how hard they've been working.

Intensity is far more important than volume. You're going to maintain the same volume—12 to 30 minutes—throughout the

REPS	WORK ZONE	REST ZONE
1	12 min./Z1	n/a
1	20 min./Z1	n/a
1	30+ min./Z1	n/a
3	2 min./Z2	2 min./Z1
2	3 min./Z2	3 min./Z1
2	4 min./Z2	3 min./Z1
2	5 min./Z2	3 min./Z1
4	30 sec./Z3	1 min./Z1
4	1 min./Z3	2 min./Z1
10	15 sec./Z3	30 sec./Z1
4	1½ min./Z3	1½ min./Z1

program, but you'll ratchet up the intensity as you go along.

Don't feel limited to gym equipment. If you'd rather do your ESD work by sprinting up hills, biking, or even swimming, then by all means go for it. You might, however, want to purchase a heart-rate monitor; $50 buys a pretty good one. (For information on specific products and recommendations, please consult www.coreperformance.com.) Keep in mind that the transition from doing your cardio work outside and your other units inside could add some time to your workout.

If you're already a serious endurance athlete, *Core Performance* is still for you. Incorporate our other units into your program, including Regeneration, and apply these ESD concepts into your existing training schedule.

On the other hand, if you're trying to gain weight, you'll want to minimize ESD work and focus more on the Elasticity and Strength units. And those who are pressed for time and forced to cut back somewhere in this program should focus on the six other Core units and skip this one. You're still getting an ESD benefit.

ESD routines will vary throughout the program. The variables are the amount of time spent in each zone and the recovery time between reps. As you advance, you'll spend more time in zones 2 and 3.

A 15-minute routine could look like this:

- A 3-minute warmup in zone 1.
- One set of the following: 2 minutes in zone 2, then 2 minutes in zone 1. If that set contains three reps, you have 12 minutes. With the 3-minute warmup, that's 15 minutes.

If calculating heart-rate zones and dealing with heart-rate monitors seems a bit much for you, then try to define three different zones for yourself. Think of zone 3 as maximum effort, zone 2 as being too intense to carry a conversation, and zone 1 as moderate enough to chat.

The key is to maximize your effort and to keep redefining your zones as your work capacity increases.

SUMMARY: Unlike traditional cardio work, Energy System Development focuses on quality, not quantity, and trains the lactate, alactate, and aerobic systems. ESD improves the function of the entire cardiovascular system while building endurance and helping the body tap into new energy levels.

TIME CAPSULE: You will work on ESD formally two or three times a week. But if you're working at a fast pace and high intensity in the other units of the Core Workout, you'll be receiving a similar benefit—even if you're too pressed for time to do ESD work.

MARY PIERCE

PROFESSIONAL TENNIS PLAYER
DATE OF BIRTH: 1/15/75

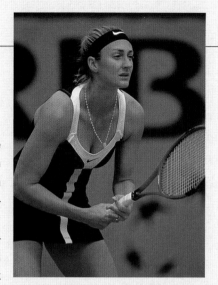

ON ESD AND TAPPING INTO ENERGY RESERVES

There's a picture of me hanging on the wall in the conference room adjacent to Mark Verstegen's office at Athletes' Performance. I'm in a black sports bra and shorts, sweating and twisting my torso with a medicine ball in my hands. The photo was taken for an advertisement, and I'm clearly in the best shape of my life.

It was about that time that I experienced perhaps the most memorable moment of my career, winning the 2000 French Open in Paris. I defeated Conchita Martinez in the final, but the match that stands out most was the semifinal against Martina Hingis, who at the time was the top-ranked player on the tour.

Martina managed to tie the match by winning the second set, 7–5. After that set, I was dog-tired, and my muscles were cramping. I wondered how I would play the decisive third set, let alone beat Martina.

Something made me think of the killer workouts I had done with Mark, in which he pushed me further than I believed I could possibly go. It seemed as if we took the most strenuous elements of the Core Workout and tried to do them as quickly as possible. I thought of that workout and others like it, and it was almost as if I could hear Mark's motivating voice in my head.

Mark spends a lot of time emphasizing "energy system development," which you might think of as cardio. The idea behind it is that you can develop energy to tap into during the highest levels of physical stress.

This clearly was one of those times. During the break, I looked over at Martina and thought, "If I'm tired, imagine what she must be feeling." That's no knock on her; it's just I knew what I was capable of, having gone through some grueling ESD workouts with Mark.

I overcame the stress to win the final set, 6–2. The following day, I teamed with Martina to win the doubles championship. The day after that, I won the singles title. So much for being cramped and tired. My ESD training with Mark gave me a mental and physical toughness to fight through the fatigue and perform at my best.

I've always been a big believer in the mind/body connection. I know I'm happier and more confident in myself when I like what I see in the mirror. That same confidence plays a huge role in how you feel about yourself mentally and emotionally.

That alone is a powerful thing. But when you combine it with the mental strength that comes from knowing that you can perform at your best even during times of stress, then you'll develop a confidence that you can deal with anything.

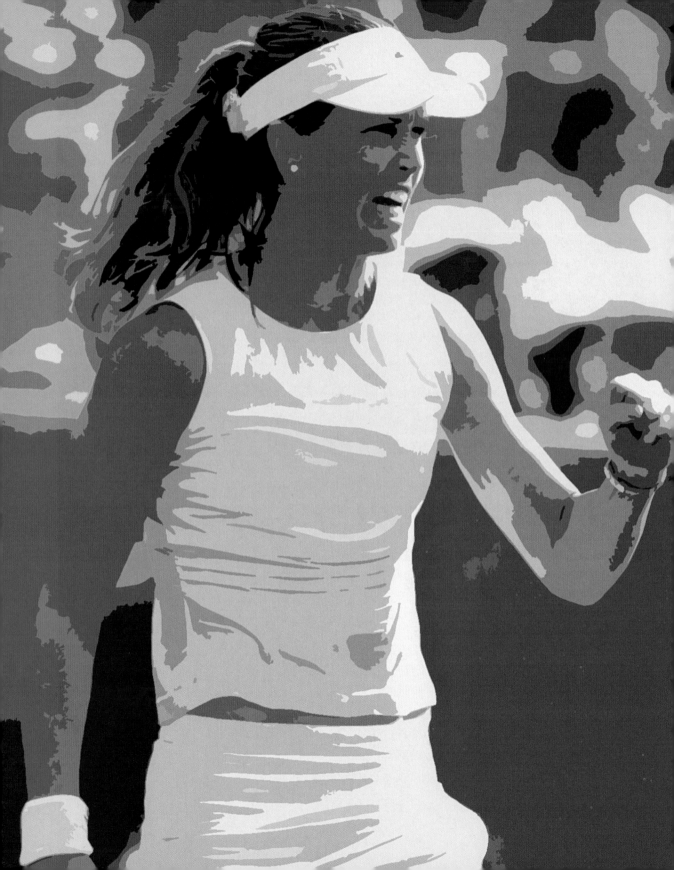

CHAPTER 11

REGENERATION

M ost fitness programs take an all-or-nothing approach. When you're training, you train very hard. And when you aren't training, you do nothing. No matter the circumstances, you do it all or you do nothing.

The problem with that formula is that it fails to facilitate one of the most important aspects of training: the repair of muscles and cells. If you're sore from a workout, for example, you have two bad choices: Go out and give yourself an equally brutal workout, or do nothing.

In truth, you need to combine quality work with quality rest to get the results you want.

The Regeneration or "reloading" section of the Core Workout, like the other units, is a series of exercises. But regeneration is also a lifestyle philosophy, a recognition that you need to plan ways to recover—mentally and physically—in all areas of your life. You experience the benefit of work on the days you rest.

There's a big difference between rest—doing nothing at all—and "active rest." In the latter, you take a break from serious training but still do things that benefit your body, such as playing golf, tennis, or basketball. Wednes-

days and Saturdays are lighter days of the Core Workout, so you might use those days, and/or Sundays, to play your favorite sport. You're not training per se, but you're still getting the benefit of physical activity. Not only that, you're having fun.

We call it *active* recovery, because you're making a modest effort. There's also *passive* recovery, which includes getting a massage and sitting in a hot tub or a cold plunge. Both elements of recovery are not only important but also necessary. And not only necessary, but equally important as working out. If you don't give your body time to recover, it's never going to improve.

You're going to train on 2 or 3 designated regeneration days, but it's going to be low stress, both physically and mentally, so your body can recover from the rigors of the other days.

You can do the Regeneration unit at home,

CORE LIFE PRINCIPLE: REGENERATION
WORK + REST = SUCCESS

Just as regeneration is crucial for the body to experience the gains it made by working out, it's important that we take time to "regenerate" or "reload" in all aspects of life. The time spent at rest is when we enjoy the fruits of our labor, when we realize the gains produced by all of our hard work. Not only that, but we recharge our batteries and come back invigorated and stronger, ready to perform at even higher levels.

Unlike many European countries, where workers typically have 4 to 6 weeks of summer vacation, we tend to work too much in the United States, even skipping vacations. But if you're working all the time, you're never truly recovered. You might think you're working hard, but you're so mentally and physically fatigued that you're not nearly as productive as you think you are. If you work all the time and don't have a chance to enjoy what you've worked for, what's the point? Apply a pattern of rest and regeneration to balance all aspects of your life, and you'll be amazed at how high the quality of your life becomes.

CORE LIFE ACTION: What activities help you regenerate and reload? Take a minute or two right now to list a few of them.

much of it while watching television, if you want. I want you to think of *Core Performance* as something that you incorporate into your entire lifestyle, not just when you eat or exercise. So just as you might do some Movement Prep exercises after you've been sitting on a plane or in a meeting for hours, you could do Regeneration exercises while watching a ball game or catching up on the day's stock-market news.

People tend to measure how effectively they've worked out by how sore they are the following days. But what good is a workout that leaves you so sore that you can't work out for the next 4 days?

Some people talk about how they train "all out" or "give 110 percent" every time they swipe their card at the gym. But let's face facts: First, they're lying; no one can work out like that without breaking down. They might do 110 percent of what the guy on the next bench is capable of doing, but they can't push themselves to their own limits without their bodies breaking down. Second, if they really try to exert that kind of effort every time they work out, they aren't training very efficiently. What people don't realize is that their bodies improve and adapt to stress on regeneration days, when they're recovering from the high-intensity days.

TAKING THE PLUNGE ■

Scandinavians have long understood the value of what we at Athletes' Performance call hot and cold contrasts. You've probably seen video of people in Sweden or Finland dashing out of a sauna or hot tub in the middle of winter and standing in the cold, if not diving into a snowbank or ice-cold pond. Some might be doing it for kicks or to join some "Polar Bear" club, but most do it because they've discovered the health benefits of contrasting hot and cold temperatures.

When you're sweating profusely in a sauna, hot tub, or bath, the blood rushes away from your internal organs and toward your skin in an attempt to keep your most vital working parts from overheating. As a result, your skin turns red.

On the other hand, if you jump into a pool of cold water, the blood rushes away from your skin to keep your internal organs safe and warm. When this happens, you tend to lose color.

In other words, hot and cold contrasts force your blood to move fast, from your organs to your skin and back again. That's a good thing in and of itself, as is exercise. But when you do it immediately after a workout, you stimulate muscle recovery with hardly any effort. The cold therapy, in particular, decreases the natural postworkout inflammation in your muscles. (Hard resistance exercise creates tiny microtears in muscle fibers, which your body repairs in between workouts, leaving your muscles bigger and stronger.)

Admittedly, there's a degree of discomfort to plunging, but I prefer to look at it as a metaphor for life. You need to get out of your comfort zone, avoid complacency, and try new things to grow and progress. As in life, it's important to remember that this discomfort and pain will pass.

Alternate between 2 to 3 minutes in a hot tub and 30 seconds to 1 minute in a cold plunge. Do this three or four times for maximum benefit. This also is a good time to drink a postworkout recovery shake, or even a glass of water.

You don't need access to a hot tub or cold plunge; you can get the same effect in the shower by switching between hot and cold settings. In fact, think of the shower as your standard equipment and having access to a hot tub or cold plunge as an added bonus.

If it's at the end of the day, you might want to finish the session in the hot setting. But if it's early, or if you need energy for the evening, end with cold. You'll find it's invigorating, keeping you alert for hours.

There's no excuse not to do this. You have to take a shower anyway, so it doesn't take any additional time. You jump-start your recovery process, and you don't even have to jump in a snowbank!

The better and more rapidly you recover, the more quickly your body adapts, and the sooner you can do another high-intensity activity. That means better gains and faster improvements. Regeneration, in other words, could be the difference between reaching and not reaching your goals.

Here's why: If you just sit on the couch or

at your desk all day, your body's systems are stagnant, like a pool of water. But if you're doing light exercise on those Regeneration days, you're increasing circulation. That pumping blood drives nutrients into your muscles, accelerating the recovery process. You can do this without high-impact activities. All you need to do is move enough to increase circulation, and move purposefully enough to activate the nervous system and elongate muscles. There's no need to stress muscles and joints; all they need is for you to flip the "on" switch.

Regeneration also is vital from a mental standpoint. If I have you train hard 6 days a week and challenge your endurance and confidence every day, you're going to burn out. Even our pro athletes would drop out. But if you know there are 2 or 3 days a week when you can relax a bit, you'll not only look forward to those days but also be inspired to work harder on the more difficult training days.

In a sense, Regeneration is incorporated throughout the Core Workout. When you consume a preworkout "shooter" or postworkout recovery shake—which will be explained in chapter 13—you're helping your body bounce back. When you're getting adequate sleep, keeping alcohol in moderation, and eating properly, you're helping the recovery process.

The Regeneration unit requires some inexpensive items: a foam roll and an 8-foot length of rope. The roll is an 18-inch-long roll of tightly packed foam that's roughly 5 inches in diameter. (In a pinch, you also could use a basketball.) On Regeneration days, you'll rotate and roll your hamstrings, quadriceps, back, lats, and hips over the foam roll.

The foam-roll routine is like a massage. It uses deep compression to help roll out the muscle spasms that develop over time. The compression causes the nerves to relax and also loosens muscle, gets the blood flowing, and helps the body recover. Think of your body as clay. The roll softens up the clay so you can remold it into something more pliable and functional.

You'll probably enjoy the foam-roll routine—everyone likes massages. Still, there'll be some uncomfortable moments, as there would be during a professional massage. Once you're past the first few weeks, though, it'll get considerably easier and more comfortable. The foam roll is a great barometer of the quality of your muscle and connective tissue. The better it feels, and the less it hurts, the higher the quality of your tissue.

Feel free to work with the foam roll on non-regeneration days; it's easy to do while watching television. Don't limit yourself to the areas targeted in this program. Use it anywhere you feel tight and in need of a massage. Foam rolls are inexpensive and available at www.coreperformance.com.

The other component of the Regeneration

A *REALLY* GOOD NIGHT'S SLEEP ■

Throughout this program, I want you to make the best use of your time and get the most benefit, whether it's working out, eating, or even sleeping. You probably know to get 8 hours of sleep a night. But you might not know that it's possible to improve the quality of your sleep by thinking in terms of 90-minute cycles.

The longer you're asleep, the longer you experience rapid-eye-movement (REM) sleep, a period marked by increased brain activity and muscle relaxation. Not surprisingly, people tend to dream during REM sleep.

Sleep cycles last approximately 90 minutes. At the end of each cycle, you start to come out of sleep. Like the groundhog that rises up to look for his shadow, your body senses whether or not it can go into another sleep cycle.

If you're awakened in the middle of a sleep cycle by an alarm clock or dream, you tend to be disoriented and end up feeling sluggish for much of the day. But if you can manage to wake up at the top of a 90-minute cycle, you'll feel more alert and invigorated.

You'll need to experiment to get the timing down, but it's not that hard once you realize how long it generally takes you to fall asleep. You should be able to better pinpoint the time and fall asleep more quickly because of your workouts, nutrition, and regeneration techniques learned in this program.

As in the Core Workout and the Core Nutrition Plan, quality is more important than quantity. Sleeping 6 hours might feel more restful than 7 hours if you get up at the top of a sleep cycle. Ideally, you'll aim for 7½ to 8 hours. But since many people struggle to get 6 hours of sleep, let's recognize that 6 hours of sleep can be a good thing—provided it's 6 hours of quality sleep, not including time spent falling asleep. Incidentally, alcohol has a negative impact on sleep.

Contrary to popular belief, you can't "catch up on your sleep." One restful night's sleep can leave you feeling refreshed and invigorated, but all those nights of missed sleep have a negative impact over time.

If you can, try to work a daily nap into your routine; a quick snooze—25 to 30 minutes—is a great way to rejuvenate yourself. Obviously, this nap is less than a 90-minute sleep cycle. But you'll awaken before you reach that deep sleep, and essentially trick your body into thinking it woke up from a REM cycle.

A few years ago, researchers studied a group of college students who were not allowed to sleep at night; instead, they took naps of 25 to 30 minutes every 4 hours, around the clock. The students were able to get by for nearly a month before collapsing.

I'm not suggesting you attempt this. But it does illustrate the restorative power of naps—and how it's possible to make the most of your time, even while asleep.

---

unit is Active-Isolated Stretching (AIS). This will require an 8- to 10-foot length of rope, about the thickness of a jump rope. If your gym doesn't have stretching ropes, you can go to a hardware store and have them cut you off a length for just a few dollars. (Or check out our ropes at www.coreperformance.com.)

Remember my anecdote about my coauthor Pete Williams earlier in the book? Pete was performing the AIS routine to loosen his hamstrings, hips, and back. He not only gained flexibility but also reprogrammed his body to remember those new ranges of motion.

You'll also recall in our discussion of Movement Prep that stretching is best done *after* a workout. (Easier to stretch a warm rubber band, right?) The AIS routine, created by Aaron Mattes (www.stretchingusa.com), is usually the last part of Regeneration, following the foam roll and a lighter version of one or two of the other units, such as Movement Prep or the Physioball Routine. (Remember, you can do all of this at home.) You might find, however, that there are times when you're feeling especially tight in an area and might want to grab a rope before or during a workout.

You'll wrap the rope around one foot at a time and perform a series of moves that will stimulate your muscles to relax and contract through new ranges of motion. You *won't* hold stretches for 10 to 30 seconds, as in traditional stretching, because that doesn't force your body to reprogram itself for new ranges of motion.

Instead, you'll use the rope to gently assist in pulling the muscle a bit farther than your body would ordinarily allow. You're going to exhale during the assistance portion, allowing a deeper stretch, then pull the leg back to the starting position.

The key is that you're reprogramming your brain. Say that you're doing a hamstring stretch. You're lying on your back, with a rope wrapped around one leg. First, you squeeze, or "fire," your quadriceps, hip flexors, and abs. As you squeeze, they contract, and your hamstrings automatically relax. That enables you to gently assist with the rope to pull your hamstrings into a slightly deeper stretch, and it helps to reprogram your brain for that new range of motion.

Since your quadriceps and hip flexors are doing the work—in these short intervals—your brain is sending signals to your quadriceps, shutting off the signals to your hamstrings, which want to resist. In a sense, you're tricking your body. Mentally, you've conditioned yourself to believe that you can stretch only to a certain point, usually because you are weak or lack coordination in that area. When you bring that hamstring back to that point, your body keeps you from moving farther. With AIS stretching, you're constantly reprogramming your body.

The great thing about the AIS routine is that people see results quickly. Remember how Pete Williams was able to go from lifting his leg 45 degrees to 90 degrees in just a matter of a few minutes? That's not uncommon. You might find it valuable to do the AIS routine daily, especially if you have a tight back or hamstrings.

SUMMARY: Regeneration is essential to recovering quickly and efficiently from exercise. The idea of Regeneration—reloading and recovering from all activities, physical and mental—needs to be incorporated into all aspects of life to obtain goals. Active recovery refers to low-intensity activity to encourage this regeneration. Passive recovery involves activities such as massage and hydrotherapy that require little to no effort.

TIME CAPSULE: Regeneration can be done at home, at work—anywhere there's an opportunity for the body to reload and recover. Though Regeneration is one of our seven units, it's more than a workout philosophy. It needs to be applied daily, weekly, monthly, and yearly to all aspects of life.

AIS COACHING KEY: To save time, do the entire series of leg stretches with one leg first, then the other. Remember to move actively through the range of motion and exhale as you gently assist with the rope. The rope should add no more than 6 to 10 percent to your range of motion.

FOAM ROLL COACHING KEY: With the foam roll, continue working an area for as long as you feel it's providing a benefit. On some days, you might feel the need for it more than on other days. Though we've limited the routine to the few examples shown, you should feel free to use it anywhere—or anytime. Many athletes find that they enjoy rolling while watching television or before bedtime. And some even like to do it before workouts, rather than after.

A CD-ROM featuring video of these exercises is available at www.coreperformance.com.

MEGHANN SHAUGHNESSY

PROFESSIONAL TENNIS PLAYER
DATE OF BIRTH: 4/17/79

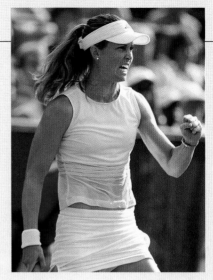

ON REST, RECOVERY, AND REGENERATION

Before I started training with Mark, I figured that if I wanted to play better, I needed to train harder. There was no time to rest if I hoped to become the best tennis player I could be. Now I understand that if I dial it down a few notches each evening and a couple of days a week, I can come back so much stronger, because I give my body a chance to recover.

The pro tennis season goes almost year-round. That's why regeneration is so important. I've come to enjoy it because it's not as if I'm doing nothing. I might ride a stationary bike, do some hot and cold contrasts, or work with a foam roll or stretching rope—all of which I can do on the road, by the way, even if it's just in the hotel gym, in my hotel room, or in the shower. Or I might do something more active, like playing basketball. Mark calls that "active rest," the idea that you're doing something that you don't think of as physical training.

Regeneration is not just a physical program. It's important to find that balance between pushing yourself as far as you can and being recovered, both physically and mentally. The most successful people find that line, where they can push themselves at the highest intensity, and know when to take a break.

That usually means taking a vacation. If you have a hectic career, that can seem impossible. But it's so important to take the time to recharge your batteries, not just 1 or 2 weeks a year but also in smaller increments each day, week, and month. Everyone has something they enjoy as a hobby that leaves them feeling refreshed. For me, it's shopping, which I like to think of as "retail therapy."

Regeneration should be a daily experience, whether it's a postworkout recovery shake, a nap, or time out to spend with family and friends.

As children, we never have to be told to do something fun. Somewhere along the way, we develop that tunnel vision of constantly working harder. There's nothing wrong with a strong work ethic, but if you never take the time to step away, you're going to burn out.

I'm lucky in that I get to do what I love for a living. That said, my profession has a high rate of burnout. If I hadn't adopted Mark's regeneration philosophies, my body definitely would have broken down. Some players have gotten so sick of tennis that they've taken leaves of absence or quit altogether.

It's funny. There was a time when I would have thought I'd be the last person Mark would ask to talk about Regeneration. But I've come to realize that it's important not just because it makes life more enjoyable but also because when you take the time to rest and recover, you come back stronger than you would have thought possible.

AIS ROPE STRETCH: STRAIGHT-LEG HAMSTRING

UNIT:
Regeneration/Flexibility.

OBJECTIVE:
To improve hamstring flexibility.

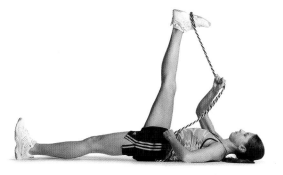

STARTING POSITION:
Lie supine (on your back) on the floor or on a table with the rope wrapped around your forefoot (see inset).

PROCEDURE:
Actively flex (squeeze) your quadriceps and hip flexors as you pull the rope back. At the end of the range of motion, exhale and slightly assist the stretch by gently pulling on the rope until you feel the stretch. Hold for 2 seconds. Inhale as you return to the starting position.

COACHING KEY(S):
Maintain quadriceps contraction. Keep your working leg straight and the opposite leg on the floor/table. Keep your working ankle "dorsiflexed," with the toes pointed up toward the shins. (The opposite movement is "plantarflexion," in which your toes are pointed.)

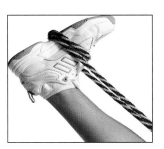

YOU SHOULD FEEL IT:
In your hamstrings and calves.

AIS ROPE STRETCH: CALF

UNIT:
Regeneration/Flexibility.

OBJECTIVE:
To improve flexibility in your calves.

STARTING POSITION:
Lie supine on the floor or on a table with the rope wrapped around your forefoot.

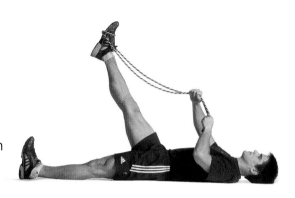

PROCEDURE:
Same procedure as with the previous hamstring stretch, but instead of bringing your leg up, pull forward toward the shin, stretching the calf for 2 seconds by slightly assisting the stretch with the rope. Exhale for a two count.

COACHING KEY(S):
Pull your toe toward your shin.

YOU SHOULD FEEL IT:
In your calves.

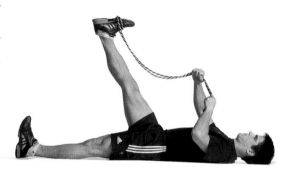

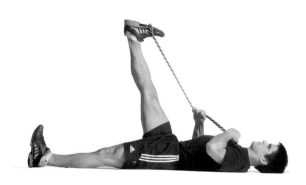

AIS ROPE STRETCH: IT/GLUTE

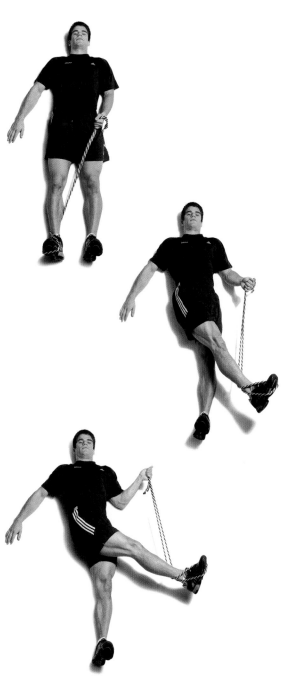

UNIT:
Regeneration/Flexibility.

OBJECTIVE:
To improve flexibility in your glutes and IT (iliotibial) bands.

STARTING POSITION:
Lie supine on the floor or on a table with a rope fastened around your foot, wrapped around the outside of your ankle, and looped underneath your leg. Hold the rope with the hand opposite the leg you're stretching. The other hand stays flat on the ground.

PROCEDURE:
While keeping the nonworking leg stationary, its toes pointed toward the ceiling, fire the adductors (the inner thigh muscles) of the working leg as you pull it across your body as far as possible. When you reach the point of resistance, give the rope a gentle assist while exhaling for 2 seconds.

COACHING KEY(S):
Fire the groin/inner thigh area (adductors) so you're able to stretch the IT bands and glutes. Keep the toes of both feet pointed toward the ceiling. Keep only your one hand on the rope, the other flat on the ground.

YOU SHOULD FEEL IT:
In the outer part of your glute and your outer thigh.

AIS ROPE STRETCH: ADDUCTORS

UNIT:
Regeneration/Flexibility.

OBJECTIVE:
To improve flexibility in your groin/inner thigh (adductor) area.

STARTING POSITION:
Lie supine on the floor or on a table with a rope fastened around your foot, wrapped around the inside of your ankle, and looped underneath your leg. Hold the rope with the hand on the same side as your working leg.

PROCEDURE:
While keeping the nonworking leg stationary, fire your glute as you sweep your leg away from your body while inhaling. When you reach the point of resistance, give the rope a gentle pull. Assist the stretch by exhaling for 2 seconds.

COACHING KEY(S):
The toes of both legs should remain pointed toward the ceiling.

YOU SHOULD FEEL IT:
In your inner thigh.

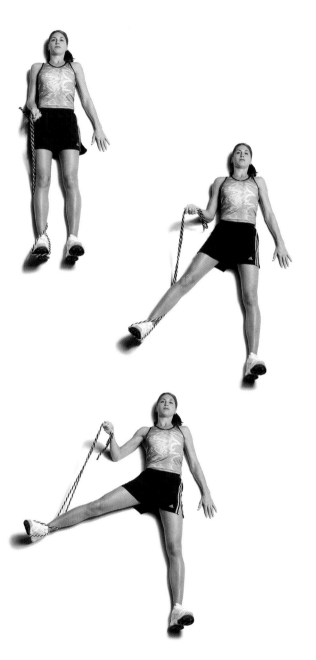

AIS ROPE STRETCH: QUAD/HIP

UNIT:
Regeneration/Flexibility.

OBJECTIVE:
To improve flexibility in your quads and hips.

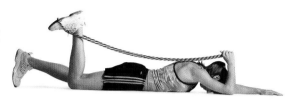

STARTING POSITION:
Lie on your stomach so that the non-working leg is straight and resting on the floor. The rope is wrapped around the foot of your working leg.

PROCEDURE:
Grab the rope over your shoulder and pull your working leg upward. Fire your glute and hamstring muscles to stretch your quad and hip. Pull your heel toward the opposite glute, much like in the scorpion exercise you learned in the Movement Prep unit.

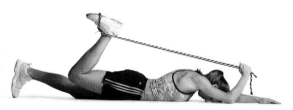

COACHING KEY(S):
Be sure to fire your hamstring and glute to get your leg back.

YOU SHOULD FEEL IT:
In your hips and the fronts of your quads.

AIS ROPE STRETCH: TRICEPS

UNIT:
Regeneration/Flexibility.

OBJECTIVE:
To improve flexibility in your triceps and rotator cuffs.

STARTING POSITION:
Take the rope in your right hand and put the hand behind your neck so that your elbow is pointed up.

PROCEDURE:
Take your left hand behind your lower back and grab the rope, palm facing out, pulling the top arm. (*Note:* If you're already flexible in this area, you might be able to clasp your hands together on one side, possibly both, and not use the rope at all.)

COACHING KEY(S):
Actively reach down the spine, exhaling to assist the stretch.

YOU SHOULD FEEL IT:
In your triceps, lats, and fronts of your shoulders.

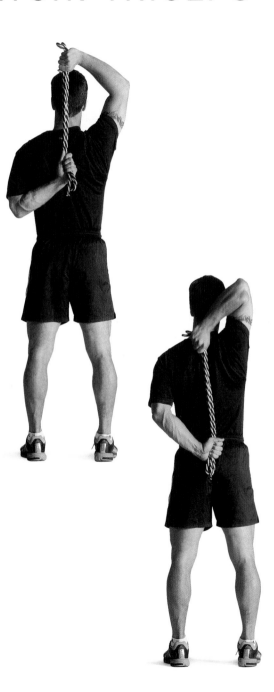

160

AIS PHYSIOBALL:
REACH, ROLL, AND LIFT

UNIT:

Regeneration/Flexibility.

OBJECTIVE:

To develop upper-back and shoulder flexibility.

STARTING POSITION:

Kneel behind a physioball with your arms extended palms up on the ball.

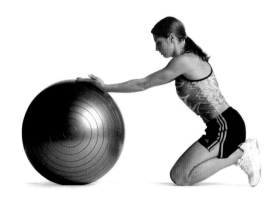

PROCEDURE:

Roll the ball forward and your hips backward as your chest drops toward the floor. Attempt to lift your hands off the ball as you exhale at the end of the stretch.

COACHING KEY(S):

Roll *the ball* forward. Don't roll forward on the ball.

YOU SHOULD FEEL IT:

In your upper back and shoulders.

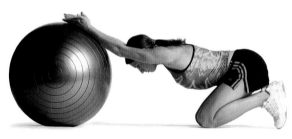

AIS 90/90 STRETCH

UNIT:
Regeneration/Flexibility.

OBJECTIVE:
To improve the flexibility of your torso rotators, which are necessary to disassociate your shoulders and hips.

STARTING POSITION:
Lie on your side, with your right leg extended and your left knee at your chest. Use your adductors (inner thigh muscles) to push your left knee to the ground, assisting with your right arm.

PROCEDURE:
Open your shoulders by rotating your torso to the left. Try to get your back and left arm flat on the ground.

COACHING KEY(S):
Keep both knees down in their starting position. Reach to get your topside shoulder flat on the ground.

YOU SHOULD FEEL IT:
In the top of your hip, your lower and mid-back, and often all the way through your chest.

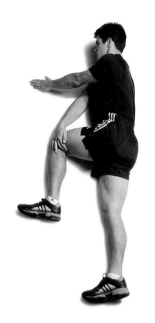

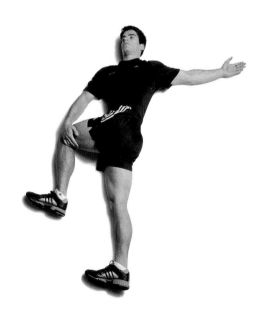

AIS QUADRUPED ROCKING

UNIT:
Regeneration/Flexibility.

OBJECTIVE:
To improve lumbar (lower-back) mobility and lengthen the muscles around your pelvis and lower back.

STARTING POSITION:
Get down on all fours and let your lower back sag.

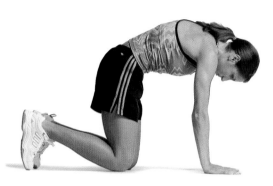

PROCEDURE:
Push your hips backward as far as you can. If your pelvis rounds under, you've gone too far.

COACHING KEY(S):
Be sure to hold your lumbar arch as you push your hips back.

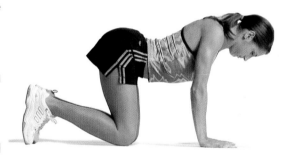

YOU SHOULD FEEL IT:
You may feel the stretch in and around your hips.

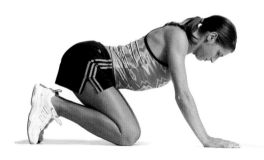

AIS SHOULDER (SIDE-LYING)

UNIT:
Regeneration/Flexibility.

OBJECTIVE:
To stretch the external-rotator muscles of your shoulder.

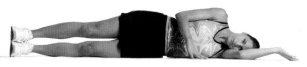

STARTING POSITION:
Lie on your side, with your bottom arm flat on the floor and your elbow bent 90 degrees.

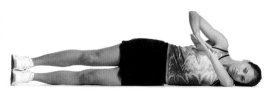

PROCEDURE:
Lower your bottom hand toward the floor in front of your belly button, gently assisting the stretch with your top arm, as shown.

COACHING KEY:
Make sure your bottom shoulder blade does not move.

YOU SHOULD FEEL IT:
In the back of your shoulder.

FOAM HAMSTRING

Place the foam roll under one or both of your hamstrings and let your body glide up and down the roll. For added benefit, try to put all your body weight on the roll. Hold perfect posture throughout.

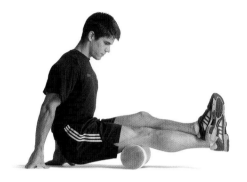

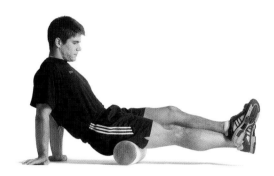

FOAM IT BAND

This might seem a little uncomfortable, but it's very effective. The iliotibial (IT) band is a thick band of tissue that extends from your hip down over your knee and attaches to your tibia (shinbone). Lie on your side and roll along the foam from your thigh to just above your knee. For greater pressure on your IT bands, stack your legs, as shown in the right photo.

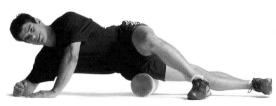

BASIC

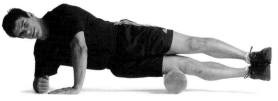

ADVANCED

FOAM QUAD

To work your quadriceps, you'll need to get on top of the foam and roll over the quads—either one at a time or both at once. You'll be surprised at how effective this particular roll is in working out muscle spasms.

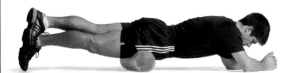 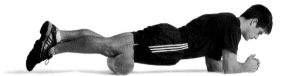

FOAM GROIN

Lie on your stomach, with one leg lifted up toward your shoulder and the roll under that leg. Roll on the inside of your thigh, from your knee to your pelvis.

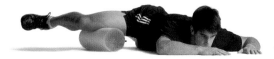 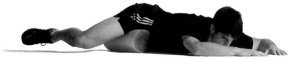

FOAM GLUTE

Sit on the foam roll and let it work from the back of your thighs to your lower back.

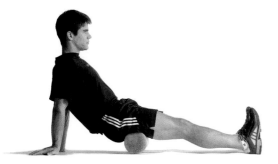 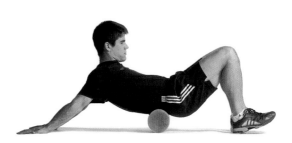

FOAM BACK

Lie atop the roll and let it glide from your shoulders down to the base of your spine. Keep your tummy tight. You can support your head with your hands, if you want.

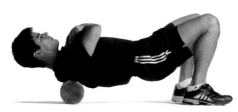 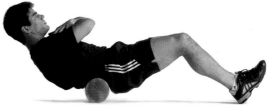

FOAM LAT

Lie on your side and roll from the side of your lower back up past your armpit.

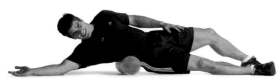 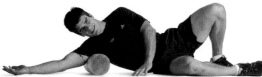

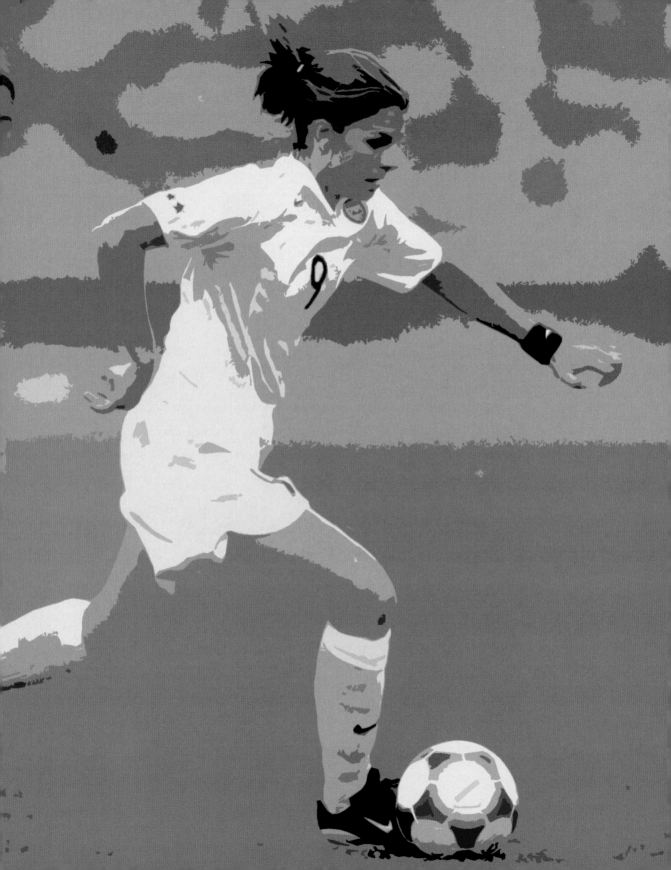

CHAPTER 12

THE CORE WORKOUT WORKSHEETS

N ow that you know what you're going to do in the Core Workout, it's time to get into the specifics of how you're going to do it. If you already skipped ahead to the worksheets that begin on page 176, you were probably bewildered by the odd nomenclature, symbols, and abbreviations. So before we go any further, let me explain how to read and use the worksheets.

Take a look at the worksheet for phase 1 on page 182. Please refer to the top row of the page, showing the week 1 indoctrination schedule, which will allow you to ease into and learn the various routines. The row below this holds the weekly schedule for weeks 2 and 3, which will be a little more challenging. Week 1 consists of a combination of Movement Prep, the Physioball Routine, Prehab, Energy System Development, Strength, and Regeneration. You do two units on Monday, Thursday, and Friday, and three on Tuesday and Wednesday. On Saturday, you do just one, and you don't do any on Sunday.

The Movement Prep, Physioball Routine, Prehab, Regeneration, and ESD exercises are listed on pages 183 to 185, along with the number of sets and reps for each. If an exercise reads "1 × 8," for instance, the reader should do one set of eight repetitions.

The @ symbol appears after some sets/reps listings. This means you should do that many reps per each leg or side of your body. This probably is self-explanatory, but the @ symbol just serves as a reminder.

In the middle of page 182, you'll notice what appears to be a complex grid. Actually, it's quite simple. It represents the Strength unit and, in the case of phase 1, is only applicable on Tuesdays and Fridays. In fact, it's used only five times over the course of phase 1: twice on Tuesdays and three times on Fridays. (It's logged in columns accordingly.)

You'll notice a series of numbers such as "212," "301," and "302," usually along the top of the Strength grid. This refers to the tempo of the lift and was devised by Ian King, an Australian strength coach. The first number refers to the number of seconds it should take you to lower the weight to start the exercise (as in a bench press) or to finish the movement if the weight starts out in the spot from which you'll lift it (as in a row or deadlift). So if the first number is 2, it should take you 2 seconds to lower the weight.

Why tell you how fast to lower a weight? Most people let the weight itself dictate its speed—you raise it slowly against the force of gravity, then lower it quickly because gravity takes over. But there's a lot of value in forcing this *eccentric* contraction to take longer. Slowing the pace forces your muscles to work harder, and harder-working muscles get bigger and stronger faster.

The second number refers to the *isometric* contraction, or the number of seconds the weight spends at the bottom before you begin to push it back up. If the middle number is 1, you pause for a full second after lowering the weight. If it's 0, you don't pause between lowering and lifting.

The third number is the speed of the actual lift, or the *concentric* contraction. It's usually 1 or 2 seconds, although in the program's later phases, you might see an "X" instead of the third number (as in 30X). This means you should lift the weight as fast and "explosively" as possible, without compromising your perfect exercise form. Even if the weight is too heavy to lift quickly, you'll still recruit more muscle fibers by trying to move it fast.

You'll see the first strength exercise listed as "Alt DB Bench Press," which stands for, of course, alternate dumbbell bench press. You'll also see a series of numbers in boxes, ranging from 10 to 15, across the row underneath the various Tuesday and Friday strength workouts. These numbers represent the prescribed number of repetitions for this exercise. Each number represents a set, and each column represents a workout. So if you see two numbers following an exercise, as there are for "Alt DB Bench Press" on Tuesday (Week 1), you should do two sets.

There's plenty of space next to the number of repetitions. This is for you to write in the amount of weight lifted. Always choose the most weight you think you can lift for the designated number of reps. If that weight proves to be too light, use a heavier one for the next set or the next workout.

You'll also notice that "Superset" is listed as a heading of the exercise row. This means that you should alternate sets of bench presses with the exercise that follows it: physioball leg curl. You should be able to jump right into that second exercise without resting, since the muscles used in the physioball leg curl are entirely different from those employed in the alternate dumbbell bench press.

Following along the grid, you'll do two sets of both one-arm, one-leg dumbbell rows and split squat/lunges, then proceed to a circuit of four exercises: physioball pushups plus; split dumbbell curls-to-presses; dumbbell pullover extensions; and physioball reach, roll, and lift. A circuit means you'll do one set of each, then go back to the top of the list and do a second set. You're using different muscles in each exercise, so you should be able to do the four exercises in the circuit quickly and efficiently. (Not all the exercises are from the Strength unit. For example, the physioball pushup plus is in the Prehab section.)

Energy System Development (ESD) work is simple in phase 1, since you're limited to the ESD 1 and ESD 2 routines. As listed on page 184, ESD 1 is simply 12 minutes exercising in zone 1, which we outlined in the ESD chapter. (You take your maximum heart rate—220 minus your age—and multiply it by 60 and 70 percent. That's your range for the entire 12 minutes.)

The ESD 2 routine, as listed near the top of page 184, is simply 20 minutes spent exercising in zone 1.

THE PHASES

The Core Workout is 12 weeks, divided into four 3-week phases. Each phase is organized on two spreadsheets. In phase 1 ("Core Foundation"), you'll learn the basics to increase mobility, stability, and balance while building an aerobic base. The first week will be light compared to the rest of the program as we get acclimated to the workout.

In phase 2 ("Extensive"), you'll turn up the intensity and amount of work. You'll add weight and reps, introduce the Elasticity routine, and pump up the volume with the ESD work.

Phase 2 will also put you into zone 2 for your ESD work. So instead of working between 60 and 70 percent of your maximum heart rate, you'll go up to 71 to 80 percent of your max. I don't expect you to maintain your heart rate in zone 2 for the duration of your workout, of course. That's why I list ESD 4, for instance, as "15 minutes/3 reps." You'll do a 3-minute warmup in zone 1, then three 4-minute reps: 2 minutes in zone 2, followed by 2 minutes in zone 1, and repeat that two more times.

In phases 3 ("Intensive") and 4 ("Mixed"), you'll increase the intensity even further, recognizing not only that you've mastered these movements but also that it's time to start generating strength and elastic power. Your body adapts quickly to exercise routines, so my goal is to challenge you continually throughout the 12 weeks.

RECOMMENDED EQUIPMENT FOR *CORE PERFORMANCE* ■

Here's what you need to get the most out of the Core Workout.

ESSENTIALS*

- Shaker bottle
- Foam roll
- Stretch rope
- Physioball

*You can pick up all these as a set at www.coreperformance.com.

IF YOU EXERCISE AT HOME

BASICS:

- Slideboard top, linoleum, tile, or hardwood exercise floor
- Dumbbells, fixed or adjustable; I highly recommend selectorized dumbbells, such as Power Blocks
- Bench that adjusts to flat or incline positions; you can purchase these and other items at www.coreperformance.com
- Aerobic steps and/or sturdy boxes that will hold your weight and withstand the impact of jumps
- Pullup bar, which can go in or over a doorway; you can also get a stand-alone station for dips and pullups

MORE SERIOUS HOME SETUP:

- Olympic barbell set with up to 300 pounds of weights
- Heavy-duty flat/incline bench with uprights for bench presses (for a bit more money, you can get uprights that go up high enough to be used as squat stands, and some benches also accommodate dip bars)

WHAT IF YOU'RE IN PAIN, DECONDITIONED, OR TIGHT?

The first workout sheet, on page 176, is the Preliminary Core Workout. It's a supplemental workout, a prequel, for people who, for whatever reason, don't feel ready to begin the standard 12-week program. Start with this program if . . .

- You're *really* out of shape, meaning you haven't worked out in years.
- You're coming off an injury-related layoff.
- You get some exercise, but your body is very tight—if you're a guy, you can't remember the last time you touched your toes.

- Squat rack, which can also be used for bench presses (you slide your own adjustable bench inside the cage) and pullups (if your ceiling is high enough)
- Cable apparatus with high and low pulleys (you can get a simple cable attachment for the back of your power cage, although you may find it difficult to do three-dimensional exercises inside the cage; in general, you won't find a cable apparatus designed for the home market that has the smooth action of a commercial machine). A Bowflex is an excellent alternative (www.bowflex.com).
- Cardio machine, such as a VersaClimber, treadmill, exercise bike, stairclimber, elliptical machine, or rower.

VERY HIGH-END HOME SETUP:

- Commercial-quality cable apparatus. Keiser equipment is recommended (www.keiser.com).
- Hot tub, cold plunge, sauna, and/or steam room

COOL OPTION FOR HOME:

- Olympic bumper plates, which are the size of 45-pound Olympic plates but come in lighter weights, such as 5, 10, or 25 pounds; these allow you to learn the most difficult lifts (such as snatches and cleans) with plates that are the right size for the lifts

HEALTH CLUB

Make sure, before you sign up for a health club, that it has the features you want, including physioballs, smoothly functioning cable machines (such as those made by Keiser), and perhaps a pool, hot tub, sauna, or even cold plunge, if those are important to you. Even if your gym has foam rolls and stretch ropes, you may prefer to bring your own for cleanliness and convenience.

You also might consider starting with this program if . . .

- You're over 40 and haven't exercised consistently in recent memory.
- You're over 50 and exercise regularly, but always at a very low intensity (walking, exercise-machine circuits at your health club, and so forth).

The 3-week Preliminary Core Workout program serves two purposes: You'll learn the basics of the Core Workout, and you'll ease into a regular exercise routine. Once you make it through those 3 weeks, I'm confident that you'll be able to start the regular program at phase 1.

If after those first 3 weeks you still feel as if you need more preparation for the full program, try the 3-week "Intermediate" workout. Once you've completed that, you should be ready to skip over phase 1 and proceed to phase 2.

You'll also note that the programs have "short" and "full" versions. Choose the one that seems most appropriate. If you need more work on one area—flexibility, say—then choose the "full" version of Regeneration, even if you choose the "short" versions of other units. Conversely, if you're deconditioned, you probably need to start with the "short" version of everything. Just remember that your goal is to be able to complete the "full" version of each unit before you get to phase 2 of the Core Workout.

HOW TO TRAIN

I want you to change your mindset about working out, not just what you're going to accomplish and your goals but also your fundamental approach to spending time in the gym.

People waste entirely too much time. They'll do a set of one exercise, stand around, get a drink of water, chat with friends, and glance at CNN before getting back to work. That's not conducive to being productive. Though having a workout partner is a good thing, both as motivation and also to serve as a spotter, it sometimes can be a distraction if you spend too much time talking and not enough time training.

I want you to become more efficient in your workouts. You might glance at these workout sheets and think, "There's no way I can get all of that done in 45 minutes or an hour." There will be a learning curve, and it might take you a few extra minutes early on. But if you're focused and work efficiently, there's no reason why you can't get a phenomenal workout in a modest amount of time.

The workout is arranged so there's little need for rest in between movements. As I explained above, I've paired many exercises in supersets so that you can proceed almost immediately from one exercise to another because the two movements work opposing muscles.

It's okay to have a workout partner, but think of that person as working alongside you, rather than trading sets with you—the partner rests while you work, and you work while the partner works. Too many people who do bodybuilding-based workout routines alternate exercises, serving as spotters for every set and effectively doubling the length of the workout.

With the exception of the bench press and maybe a few other exercises in the Core Workout, there's really no need for a spotter. You can have a workout partner—or two or three. Just do all of the exercises together at the same time.

I know it can be intimidating going to a gym, especially if you're working out differently than everyone else in the room. Just remember that what you're doing is far more efficient and beneficial than what everyone else is doing. Don't let some know-it-all person discourage you. As Nomar Garciaparra mentioned in the foreword, you'll likely have people asking you to show them a thing or two.

A few questions you may have:

Q: WHAT DO I DO AFTER I FINISH THE CORE WORKOUT?

A: Of course, I don't want you to stop at the end of 12 weeks. You can continue the phase 4 program for a few weeks, increasing the amount of weight you use. We'll also provide advanced Core Workout routines on our Web site: www.coreperformance.com.

Q: WHAT DO I DO WHEN I CAN'T FIT IN AN ENTIRE WORKOUT?

A: Obviously, there will be times when work, travel, and family commitments make it impossible to get in an entire workout. The important thing is to do something. Instead of beating yourself up about not doing a full workout, give yourself credit for getting something done in spite of the obstacles.

With that in mind, I've included an abbreviated version of the Core Workout on page 198 that can be done in a hotel room or if you're otherwise pressed for time and/or lack facilities. You'll note that I've preserved the sequence of our seven units—Movement Prep, Prehab, Physioball Routine, Elasticity, Strength, ESD, and Regeneration. Feel free to move ESD to the beginning or end of the workout, but try to keep the others in order to get the maximum physiological response.

Since you're pressed for time, you're only going to be working through a few units. But maintain the order. If you're going to perform, say, Movement Prep, Prehab, and Elasticity, do them in that order to get the most benefit.

PRELIMINARY CORE WORKOUT

Pain, Deconditioned, or Tight? Start Here!

MONDAY	TUESDAY	WEDNESDAY
Regeneration: Foam	Regeneration: AIS	Regeneration: Foam
Movement Prep	Regeneration: Foam	Movement Prep
Regeneration: AIS	Physioball	Regeneration: AIS
Strength (odd week)/Prehab (even week)	Walk/Lifestyle (sports, yard	Prehab
ESD 1 (odd week)/ESD 2 (even week)	work—whatever you enjoy	Strength (even week)
Nutrition: Shake	that keeps you moving)	Nutrition: Shake

BEGINNER Weeks 1–3

STRENGTH (GYM)

Exercise	Short (10 min.)	Full (20 min.)
SUPERSET		
Alt DB Bench Press	1 × 15	2 × 12
Floor/PB Leg Curl	1 × 15	2 × 12
SUPERSET		
1-Arm, 1-Leg DB Row	1 × 15@	2 × 12@
Split Squat/Lunge	1 × 15@	2 × 12@
SUPERSET		
Split DB Curl-to-Press	1 × 15@	2 × 12@
Floor/PB Pushup Plus	1 × 15	2 × 12

MOVEMENT PREP

Exercise	Short (5 min.)	Full (10 min.)
Hip Crossover (feet flat)	8@	6@
Scorpion	—	6@
Calf Stretch	—	6@
Hand Walk	4	6
Inverted Hamstring	—	6@
Forward Lunge/Forearm-to-Instep	4@	6@
Backward Lunge with a Twist	—	6@
Drop Lunge	—	6@
Lateral Lunge	4@	6@
Sumo Squat-to-Stand	8	6

THURSDAY	FRIDAY	SATURDAY
Regeneration: AIS	Regeneration: Foam	Regeneration: AIS/Foam (optional)
Regeneration: Foam	Movement Prep	Physioball
Physioball	Regeneration: AIS	Walk/Lifestyle
Walk/Lifestyle	Strength (odd week)/Prehab (even week)	Nutrition: Shake
	ESD 2 (odd week)/ESD 1 (even week)	
	Nutrition: Shake	

PREHAB

Exercise	Short (5 min.)	Full (10 min.)
Floor/PB *Y*	8	12
Floor/PB *T*	8	12
Floor/PB *W*	8	12
Floor/PB *L*	8	12
Floor/PB Pushup Plus	8	12
PB Reach, Roll, and Lift	—	12
Glute Bridge w/Adduction	8	12
Quadruped Circles	—	12@
Pillar Bridge Front	20 sec.	30 sec.
Pillar Bridge Side (right/left)	8@	12@

REGENERATION

Exercise	Short (7 min.)	Full (12 min.)
Foam Hamstring	1 × 8@	1 × 10@
Foam IT Band	1 × 8@	1 × 10@
Foam Quad/Groin	1 × 8@	1 × 10@
Foam Glute	1 × 8	1 × 10
Foam Back/Lat	—	1 × 10@
AIS Rope Calf	—	1 × 10@
AIS Rope Hamstring	1 × 8@	1 × 10@
AIS Rope IT/Glute	1 × 8@	1 × 10@
AIS Rope Adductors	—	1 × 10@
AIS Rope Quad/Hip	1 × 8@	1 × 10@
AIS Shoulder (Side-Lying)	1 × 8@	1 × 10@
AIS Rope Triceps	—	1 × 10@
AIS 90/90 Stretch	1 × 8@	1 × 10@
AIS Quadruped Rocking	—	1 × 10

Pain, Deconditioned, or Tight? Start Here!

BEGINNER Weeks 1–3 (cont.)

PHYSIOBALL

Exercise	Short (5 min.)	Full (10 min.)
Lateral Roll	8@	12@
Russian Twist	8@	12@
Plate Crunch	8	12
Lying Opposites	—	20 sec.@
Reverse Crunch	—	12
Bridging	20 sec.	20 sec.
Hip Crossover	—	12@

ESD

Workout	Total	Work/Zone
1 Aerobic/Recovery	12 min.	12 min./Z1 Lower
2 Aerobic/Recovery	20 min.	20 min./Z1 Lower

Zone 1 = 60–70% of 220 – age

INTERMEDIATE Weeks 4–6

STRENGTH (GYM)

Exercise	Short (10 min.)	Full (20 min.)
SUPERSET		
Alt DB Bench	1×10	2×8
Split Squat/Lunge	$1 \times 10@$	$2 \times 8@$
SUPERSET		
1-Arm, 1-Leg DB Row	$1 \times 10@$	$2 \times 8@$
Floor/PB Leg Curl	1×10	2×8
CIRCUIT		
Cable Lifting	$1 \times 10@$	$2 \times 8@$
Cable Chopping	$1 \times 10@$	$2 \times 8@$
Split DB Curl-to-Press	$1 \times 5@$	$2 \times 4@$
Floor/PB Pushup Plus	1×10	2×8

MOVEMENT PREP

Exercise	Short (6 min.)	Full (12 min.)
Hip Crossover (knees bent)	6@	8@
Scorpion	—	8@
Calf Stretch	—	8@
Hand Walk	6	8
Inverted Hamstring	6@	8@
Forward Lunge/ Forearm-to-Instep	6@	8@
Backward Lunge with a Twist	6@	8@
Drop Lunge	6@	8@
Lateral Lunge	6@	8@
Sumo Squat-to-Stand	6	8

INTERMEDIATE Weeks 4–6 (cont.)

PHYSIOBALL

Exercise	Short (5 min.)	Full (10 min.)
Lateral Roll	8@	12@
Russian Twist	8@	12@
Plate Crunch	8	12
Lying Opposites	—	20 sec.
Reverse Crunch	—	12
Bridging	20 sec.	20 sec.
Hip Crossover	—	12@

REGENERATION

Exercise	Short (7 min.)	Full (12 min.)
Foam Hamstring	1 × 8@	1 × 10@
Foam IT Band	1 × 8@	1 × 10@
Foam Quad/Groin	1 × 8@	1 × 10@
Foam Glute	1 × 8	1 × 10
Foam Back/Lat	—	1 × 10@
AIS Rope Calf	—	1 × 10@
AIS Rope Hamstring	1 × 8@	1 × 10@
AIS Rope IT/Glute	1 × 8@	1 × 10@
AIS Rope Adductors	—	1 × 10@
AIS Rope Quad/Hip	1 × 8@	1 × 10@
AIS Shoulder (Side-Lying)	1 × 8@	1 × 10@
AIS Rope Triceps	—	1 × 10@
AIS 90/90 Stretch	1 × 8@	1 × 10@
AIS Quadruped Rocking	—	1 × 10

PREHAB

Exercise	Short (5 min.)	Full (10 min.)
Floor/PB *Y*	8	12
Floor/PB *T*	8	12
Floor/PB *W*	8	12
Floor/PB *L*	8	12
Floor/PB Pushup Plus	8	12
PB Reach, Roll, and Lift	—	12
Glute Bridge w/Adduction	8	12
Quadruped Circles	—	12@
Pillar Bridge Front	20 sec.	30 sec.
Pillar Bridge Side (right/left)	8@	12@

ESD

Workout	Total	Work/Zone
1 Aerobic/Recovery	12 min.	12 min./Z1 Upper
2 Aerobic/Recovery	20 min.	20 min./Z1 Upper

Zone 1 = 60–70% of 220 – age

THE CORE WORKOUT

Phase 1: Core Foundation (Weeks 1, 2, and 3)
Trained: Intermediate/Advanced
Goals: Increase mobility, stability, and balance while building an aerobic base

MONDAY (WEEK 1)	TUESDAY (WEEK 1)	WEDNESDAY (WEEK 1)
ESD 1	ESD 1	ESD 1 + Movement Prep
Movement Prep	Movement Prep + Physioball	Regeneration
MONDAY (WEEKS 2 & 3)	**TUESDAY (WEEKS 2 & 3)**	**WEDNESDAY (WEEKS 2 & 3)**
Movement Prep (10 min.)	Physioball (10 min.)	ESD 2 (20 min.)
Prehab: Hip (5 min.)	Strength (30 min.)	Movement Prep (10 min.)
Prehab: Shoulder (5 min.)	**Total Time: 40 min.**	Prehab: Core (5 min.)
Prehab: Core (5 min.)	Regeneration: AIS (12 min.)	Regeneration: Foam (10 min.)
ESD 1 (12 min.)		**Total Time: 45 min.**
Total Time: 37 min.		
Regeneration: Foam (10 min.)		

STRENGTH: 30-Second Rest between Sets
Full Range of Motion and Adhere to 212 Tempo!

Exercise		Friday (Week 1)	Tuesday (Week 2)	Friday (Week 2)	Tuesday (Week 3)	Friday (Week 3)
SUPERSET						
Alt DB Bench Press	set 1	15	12	12	10	10
	set 2	—	12	12	10	10
PB Leg Curl	set 1	10	12	10	12	12
	set 2	—	10	8	10	10
SUPERSET						
1-Arm, 1-Leg DB Row	set 1	15@	12@	12@	10@	10@
	set 2	—	12@	12@	10@	10@
Split Squat/Lunge	set 1	15@	12@	12@	10@	10@
	set 2	—	12@	12@	10@	10@
CIRCUIT						
Floor/Physioball Pushup Plus	set 1	8+	10+	12+	12+	12+
	set 2	—	8+	10+	10+	10+
Split DB Curl-to-Press	set 1	8@	6@	6@	6@	6@
	set 2	—	6@	5@	5@	5@
DB Pullover Extension	set 1	15	12	12	12	12
	set 2	—	12	10	10	10
PB Reach, Roll, and Lift	set 1	10	10	10	10	10
	set 2	—	10	10	10	10

THURSDAY (WEEK 1)	FRIDAY (WEEK 1)	SATURDAY (WEEK 1)
ESD 2	ESD 1	Regeneration
Prehab 1, 2, 3	Strength	

THURSDAY (WEEKS 2 & 3)	FRIDAY (WEEKS 2 & 3)	SATURDAY (WEEKS 2 & 3)
Physioball (10 min.)	Movement Prep (10 min.)	ESD 2 (20 min.)
Prehab: Shoulder (5 min.)	Strength (30 min.)	Regeneration: Foam (10 min.)
Prehab: Hip (5 min.)	Prehab: Core (5 min.)	Regeneration: AIS (10 min.)
ESD 1 (12 min.)	**Total Time: 45 min.**	**Total Time: 40 min.**
Total Time: 32 min.		
Regeneration: AIS (12 min.)		

MOVEMENT PREP

Exercise	Week 1	Weeks 2 & 3
Hip Crossover	1 × 8@ feet down	1 × 10@ to 90° knees
Calf Stretch	1 × 8@	1 × 10@
Hand Walk	1 × 4	1 × 5
Forward Lunge/Forearm-to-Instep	1 × 4@	1 × 5@
Backward Lunge with a Twist	1 × 4@	1 × 5@
Lateral Lunge	1 × 4@	1 × 5@
Sumo Squat-to-Stand	1 × 8	1 × 10

PREHAB

PREHAB: SHOULDER (1)	Week 1	Weeks 2 & 3
Floor/PB *T*	1 × 8	1 × 10
Floor/PB *W*	1 × 8	1 × 10
Floor/PB *L*	1 × 8	1 × 10
PB Pushup Plus	1 × 8	1 × 10
PB Reach, Roll, and Lift	1 × 8	1 × 10

PREHAB: HIP (2)	Week 1	Weeks 2 & 3
Glute Bridge	1 × 8	1 × 10
Side Lying Ad/Abduction	1 × 8@	1 × 10@

PREHAB: CORE (3)	Week 1	Weeks 2 & 3
Pillar Bridge Front	1 × 20 sec.	1 × 30 sec.
Pillar Bridge Side (right/left)	1 × 15 sec.@	1 × 20 sec.@

THE CORE WORKOUT (CONT.)

Phase 1: Core Foundation (Weeks 1, 2, and 3)
Trained: Intermediate/Advanced
Goals: Increase mobility, stability, and balance while building an aerobic base

ESD (ENERGY SYSTEM DEVELOPMENT)

Workout	Total	Work/Zone
1 Aerobic/Recovery	12 min.	12 min./Z1
2 Aerobic/Recovery	20 min.	20 min./Z1

PHYSIOBALL

Exercise	Week 1	Weeks 2 & 3
Lateral Roll	1 × 8@	1 × 10@
Russian Twist	1 × 8@	1 × 10@
Plate Crunch	1 × 8	1 × 10
Lying Opposites	1 × 8@	1 × 10@
Reverse Crunch	1 × 8	1 × 10
Bridging	1 × 8	1 × 10
Hip Crossover	1 × 8@	1 × 10@

REGENERATION (Done Anytime/Anywhere!)

Exercise	Week 1	Weeks 2 & 3
Foam Hamstring	1 × 8@	1 × 10@
Foam IT Band	1 × 8@	1 × 10@
Foam Quad/Groin	1 × 8@	1 × 10@
Foam Glute	1 × 8	1 × 10
Foam Back/Lat	1 × 8@	1 × 10@
AIS Rope Calf	1 × 8@	1 × 10@
AIS Rope Hamstring	1 × 8@	1 × 10@
AIS Rope or Static IT/Glute	1 × 8@	1 × 10@
AIS Rope Adductors	1 × 8@	1 × 10@
AIS Rope or Static Quad/Hip	1 × 8@	1 × 10@
AIS Shoulder (Side-Lying)	1 × 8@	1 × 10@
AIS Rope Triceps	1 × 8@	1 × 10@
AIS 90/90 Stretch	1 × 8@	1 × 10@
AIS Quadruped Rocking	1 × 8	1 × 10

If you're pressed for time, select the 4 AIS stretches that best target your problem areas.

THE CORE WORKOUT

Phase 2: Extensive (Weeks 4, 5, and 6)
Goals: Increase elasticity, strength, work capacity/quantity

MONDAY	TUESDAY	WEDNESDAY
Movement Prep A&B (12 min.)	Movement Prep A (6 min.)	ESD 3 (30 min.)
Prehab: Core (7 min.)	Strength A (25 min.)	Physioball (12 min.)
Prehab: Hip (7 min.)	ESD 4 (15 min.)	**Total Time: 42 min.**
Prehab: Shoulder (7 min.)	**Total Time: 46 min.**	Regeneration: Foam (6 min.)
Elasticity (10 min.)		Regeneration: AIS (12 min.)
Total Time: 43 min.		
Regeneration: Foam (7 min.)		

STRENGTH: 30-Second Rest between Sets   TEMPO: 311

STRENGTH A		Tuesday	Tuesday	Tuesday
SUPERSET				
Bench Press	set 1	8	8	8
	set 2	8	8	6
	set 3	8	6	6
Romanian Deadlift (RDL)	set 1	8	8	8
	set 2	8	8	6
	set 3	8	6	6
SUPERSET				
Split Squat/Lunge	set 1	8@	8@	8@
	set 2	8@	8@	6@
	set 3	8@	8@	6@
Pullup (horiz. to vert.)	set 1	6	8	10
	set 2	6	8	10
	set 3	6	8	10
CIRCUIT				
Cable 1-Arm Rot. Row	set 1	8@	8@	8@
	set 2	8@	8@	8@
Split DB Curl-to-Press	set 1	5@	5@	5@
	set 2	4@	4@	4@
DB Pullover Extension	set 1	10	10	10
	set 2	8	8	8

		THURSDAY	FRIDAY	SATURDAY

THURSDAY
Movement Prep A&B (12 min.)
Prehab: Core (7 min.)
Prehab: Hip (7 min.)
Prehab: Shoulder (7 min.)
Elasticity (10 min.)
Total Time: 43 min.
Regeneration: Foam (7 min.)

FRIDAY
Movement Prep B (6 min.)
Strength B (20 min.)
ESD 5 (15 min.)
Total Time: 41 min.

SATURDAY
ESD 3 (30 min.)
Physioball (12 min.)
Total Time: 42 min.
Regeneration: Foam (5+ min.)
Regeneration: AIS (5+ min.)

Full Range of Motion and Adhere to 311 Tempo!

STRENGTH B		Friday	Friday	Friday
SUPERSET				
Alt DB Bench Press	set 1	10	10	8
	set 2	10	8	8
Split Squat/Lunge	set 1	10@	10@	8@
	set 2	10@	10@	8@
SUPERSET				
1-Arm, 1-Leg DB Row	set 1	10@	10@	8@
	set 2	10@	10@	8@
Floor/PB Leg Curl	set 1	8	10	12
	set 2	8	10	12
CIRCUIT				
Cable Lifting	set 1	10@	10@	10@
	set 2	8@	8@	8@
Cable Chopping	set 1	10@	10@	10@
	set 2	8@	8@	8@
Split DB Curl-to-Press	set 1	5@	5@	5@
	set 2	4@	4@	4@

THE CORE WORKOUT (CONT.)

Phase 2: Extensive (Weeks 4, 5, and 6)
Goals: Increase elasticity, strength, work capacity/quantity

MOVEMENT PREP

MOVEMENT PREP A	Week 1	Week 2	Week 3
Forward Lunge/Forearm-to-Instep	1 × 5@	1 × 6@	1 × 7@
Backward Lunge with a Twist	1 × 5@	1 × 6@	1 × 7@
Calf Stretch	1 × 10@	1 × 12@	1 × 7@
Hand Walk	1 × 5	1 × 6	1 × 7
Inverted Hamstring	1 × 5@	1 × 6@	1 × 7@

MOVEMENT PREP B	Week 1	Week 2	Week 3
Hip Crossover	1 × 10@	1 × 12@	1 × 7@
	to 90° knees	to longer legs	to ¾ to straight legs
Scorpion	1 × 10@	1 × 12@	1 × 7@
Lateral Lunge	1 × 5@	1 × 6@	1 × 7@
Drop Lunge	1 × 5@	1 × 6@	1 × 7@
Sumo Squat-to-Stand	1 × 5	1 × 6	1 × 7

PREHAB

PREHAB: SHOULDER	Week 1	Week 2	Week 3
Floor/PB *T*	1 × 8 + weight	1 × 10 + weight	1 × 12 + weight
Floor/PB *W*	1 × 8 + weight	1 × 10 + weight	1 × 12 + weight
Floor/PB *L*	1 × 8 + weight	1 × 10 + weight	1 × 12 + weight
PB Pushup Plus	1 × 8	1 × 10	1 × 12
PB Reach, Roll, and Lift	1 × 10	1 × 12	1 × 14

PREHAB: HIP	Week 1	Week 2	Week 3
Glute Bridge with Adduction	1 × 10	1 × 12	1 × 14
Side-Lying Ad/Abduction	1 × 10@	1 × 12@	1 × 14@
Quadruped Circles	1 × 5@	1 × 6@	1 × 7@

PREHAB: CORE	Week 1	Week 2	Week 3
Pillar Bridge Front	1 × 30 sec.	1 × 45 sec.	1 × 60 sec.
Pillar Bridge Side (right/left)	1 × 30 sec.@	1 × 45 sec.@	1 × 60 sec.@

ELASTICITY

Exercise	Week 1	Week 2	Week 3
Base Side-to-Side (fast)	2 × 6 sec.	2 × 8 sec.	2 × 10 sec.
Base Rotation (fast)	2 × 6 sec.	2 × 8 sec.	2 × 10 sec.
Squat Jump	2 × 5 reps	2 × 6 reps	2 × 7 reps
Lateral Bound	2 × 3 reps@	2 × 4 reps@	2 × 4 reps@

PHYSIOBALL

Exercise	Week 1	Week 2	Week 3
Lateral Roll	1 × 10@	1 × 12@	1 × 14@
Russian Twist	1 × 10 add weight@	1 × 12 + more weight@	1 × 14 + more weight@
Plate Crunch	1 × 10 add weight	1 × 12 + more weight	1 × 14 + more weight
Knee Tuck	1 × 10	1 × 12	1 × 14
Lying Opposites	1 × 10@	1 × 12@	1 × 14@
Reverse Hyper	1 × 10	1 × 12	1 × 14
Reverse Crunch	1 × 10	1 × 12	1 × 14
Bridging	1 × 10	1 × 12	1 × 14
Hip Crossover	1 × 10@	1 × 12@	1 × 14@

ESD

Workout	Total/# Reps	Warmup	Work/Zone	Rest/Zone
4 Lactate Capacity	15 min./3 reps	3 min./Z1	2 min./Z2	2 min./Z1
5 Lactate Capacity	15 min./2 reps	3 min./Z1	3 min./Z2	3 min./Z1
3 Aerobic/Recovery	—	—	30+ min./Z1	—

REGENERATION

Exercise	Week 1	Week 2	Week 3
Foam Hamstring	1 × 8@	1 × 10@	1 × 12@
Foam IT Band	1 × 8@	1 × 10@	1 × 12@
Foam Quad	1 × 8@	1 × 10@	1 × 12@
Foam Glute	1 × 8	1 × 10	1 × 12
Foam Back	1 × 8	1 × 10	1 × 12
AIS Rope Calf	1 × 8@	1 × 10@	1 × 12@
AIS Rope Hamstring	1 × 8@	1 × 10@	1 × 12@
AIS Rope IT/Glute	1 × 8@	1 × 10@	1 × 12@
AIS Rope Adductors	1 × 8@	1 × 10@	1 × 12@
AIS Rope Quad/Hip	1 × 8@	1 × 10@	1 × 12@
AIS Rope Chest	1 × 8	1 × 10	1 × 12
AIS Rope Triceps	1 × 8@	1 × 10@	1 × 12@
AIS 90/90 Stretch	1 × 8@	1 × 10@	1 × 12@
AIS Quadruped Rocking	1 × 8	1 × 10	1 × 12

If you're pressed for time, select the 4 AIS stretches that best target your problem areas.

THE CORE WORKOUT

Phase 3: Intensive (Weeks 7, 8, and 9)
Intermediate/Advanced
Goals: Speed, Power, Strength, Quality

MONDAY	TUESDAY	WEDNESDAY
Movement Prep A (6 min.)	Movement Prep B (5 min.)	ESD 3 (30 min.)
Elasticity A (10 min.)	Elasticity B (10 min.)	Prehab: Core (10 min.)
Strength A (30 min.)	Strength B (30 min.)	**Total Time: 40 min.**
Prehab: Shoulder (5 min.)	ESD 8 (15 min.)	Nutrition: Shake
Total Time: 51 min.	**Total Time: 60 min.**	Regeneration: Foam (10 min.)
Nutrition: Shake	Nutrition: Shake	Regeneration: AIS (10 min.)

STRENGTH: 60-Second Rest between Supersets   TEMPO: 30X (Explosive)

STRENGTH A		Monday	Thursday	Monday	Thursday	Monday	Thursday
SUPERSET							
Bench Press+Plyo Pushup	set 1	5+3*	8+3*	4+3*	8+3*	3+3*	6
	set 2	5+3*	8+3*	4+3*	8+3*	3+3*	**
	set 3	5+3*	8+3*	4+3*	8+3*	3+3*	**
Pullup (add weight)	set 1	6	6	4	4	3	6
	set 2	6	6	4	4	3	**
	set 3	6	6	4	4	3	**
SUPERSET							
DB Pullover Extension	set 1	6	8	5	8	4	6
	set 2	6	8	5	8	4	**
DB Curl-to-Press	set 1	6	8	5	8	4	6
	set 2	6	8	5	8	4	**
SUPERSET							
Cable Chopping	set 1	8@	8@	6@	6@	6@	6@
	set 2	8@	8@	6@	6@	6@	6@
Cable Lifting	set 1	8@	8@	6@	6@	6@	6@
	set 2	8@	8@	6@	6@	6@	6@

*Do 3 plyo pushups after each bench press set, then rest 60 seconds, do pullups, then rest 60 seconds and repeat.

**Do maximum reps with whatever weight you used in the first workout of this phase.

		THURSDAY	FRIDAY	SATURDAY

THURSDAY	**FRIDAY**	**SATURDAY**
Movement Prep A (6 min.)	Movement Prep B (5 min.)	ESD 3 (30 min.)
Elasticity A (10 min.)	Elasticity B (10 min.)	Prehab: Core (10 min.)
Strength A (30 min.)	Strength B (30 min.)	**Total Time: 40 min.**
Prehab: Shoulder (5 min.)	ESD 9 (17 min.)	Nutrition: Shake
Total Time: 51 min.	**Total Time: 62 min.**	Regeneration: Foam (10 min.)
Nutrition: Shake	Nutrition: Shake	Regeneration: AIS (10 min.)
Regeneration: Foam (7 min.)		

Full Range of Motion and Adhere to 30X Tempo!

STRENGTH B		Tuesday	Friday	Tuesday	Friday	Tuesday	Friday
SUPERSET							Reload— Do Wednesday workout
Cable 1-Arm Rot. Row	set 1	8@	8@	6@	6@	6@	
	set 2	8@	8@	6@	6@	6@	
PB Russian Twist with weight	set 1	12@	12@	10@	10@	8@	
	set 2	12@	12@	10@	10@	8@	
SUPERSET							
Split Squat+Split Jump	set 1	6+3*	6+3*	4+3*	4+3*	3+3*	
	set 2	6+3*	6+3*	4+3*	4+3*	3+3*	
PB Plate Crunch	set 1	12	12	10	10	8	
	set 2	12	12	10	10	8	
SUPERSET							
DB Front Squat+Press+Squat Jump	set 1	8+4**	8+4**	6+4**	6+4**	4+4**	
	set 2	8+4**	8+4**	6+4**	6+4**	4+4**	
PB Lateral Roll	set 1	12@	12@	10@	10@	8@	
	set 2	12@	12@	10@	10@	8@	
SUPERSET							
Romanian Deadlift (RDL)	set 1	8	6	6	6	6	
	set 2	8	6	6	6	6	
PB Prone Knee Tuck	set 1	8	8	10	10	12	
	set 2	8	8	10	10	12	

*Do 3 split jumps after each set of 6 split squat lunges, then immediately do PB plate crunches.
** Do 4 squat jumps after each set of 8 DB front squat/presses, then immediately do PB lateral rolls.

THE CORE WORKOUT (CONT.)

Phase 3: Intensive (Weeks 7, 8, and 9)
Intermediate/Advanced
Goals: Speed, Power, Strength, Quality

MOVEMENT PREP

MOVEMENT PREP A	Week 1	Week 2	Week 3
Forward Lunge/Forearm-to-Instep	1 × 5@	1 × 6@	1 × 7@
Backward Lunge with a Twist	1 × 5@	1 × 6@	1 × 7@
Calf Stretch	1 × 10@	1 × 12@	1 × 14@
Hand Walk	1 × 5	1 × 6	1 × 7
Inverted Hamstring	1 × 5@	1 × 6@	1 × 7@

MOVEMENT PREP B	Week 1	Week 2	Week 3
Hip Crossover	1 × 10@ to 90° knees	1 × 12@ to longer legs	1 × 14@ to straight legs
Scorpion	1 × 10@	1 × 12@	1 × 14@
Lateral Lunge	1 × 5@	1 × 6@	1 × 14@
Drop Lunge	1 × 5@	1 × 6@	1 × 14@
Sumo Squat-to-Stand	1 × 5	1 × 6	1 × 7
Prehab Hip: Glute Bridge (1 leg)	1 × 10@	1 × 12@	1 × 14@

PREHAB

PREHAB: SHOULDER	Week 1	Week 2	Week 3
PB Y	1 × 10 + weight	1 × 12 + weight	1 × 12 + weight
PB T	1 × 10 + weight	1 × 12 + weight	1 × 12 + weight
PB W	1 × 10 + weight	1 × 12 + weight	1 × 12 + weight
PB L	1 × 10 + weight	1 × 12 + weight	1 × 12 + weight

PREHAB: CORE	Week 1	Week 2	Week 3
Pillar Bridge Front	2 × 20 sec.	2 × 30 sec.	2 × 40 sec.
Pillar Bridge Side (right/left) Top Leg	2 × 20 sec.	2 × 30 sec.	2 × 40 sec.
Pillar Bridge Side (right/left) Bottom Leg	2 × 20 sec.	2 × 30 sec.	2 × 40 sec.

ELASTICITY

ELASTICITY A	Week 1	Week 2	Week 3
1 Leg over the Line	2 × 5 sec.	2 × 7 sec.	2 × 7 sec.
Get-Up	4 reps	5 reps	6 reps
Side-to-Side Jump-to-Sprint	2 × 4 jumps each side	3 × 5 jumps each side	4 × 6 jumps each side
ELASTICITY B	Week 1	Week 2	Week 3
Lateral Bound	2 × 5@	2 × 6@	2 × 7@
3-Hurdle Drill	3 × 8 sec.	4 × 8 sec.	4 × 10 sec.

ESD

Workout	Total/# Reps	Warmup	Work/Zone	Rest/Zone
8 Lactate Power	15 min./4 reps/2 sets	3 min./Z1	30 sec./Z3	1 min./Z1
9 Lactate Power	15 min./4 reps	3 min./Z1	1 min./Z3	2 min./Z1
3 Aerobic/Recovery	—	—	30+ min./Z1	—

REGENERATION (Done Anytime/Anywhere!)

Exercise	Week 1	Week 2	Week 3
Foam Hamstring	1 × 8@	1 × 10@	1 × 12@
Foam IT Band	1 × 8@	1 × 10@	1 × 12@
Foam Quad/Groin	1 × 8@	1 × 10@	1 × 12@
Foam Glute	1 × 8	1 × 10	1 × 12
Foam Back/Lat	1 × 8@	1 × 10@	1 × 12@
AIS Rope Calf	1 × 8@	1 × 10@	1 × 12@
AIS Rope Hamstring	1 × 8@	1 × 10@	1 × 12@
AIS Rope or Static IT/Glute	1 × 8@	1 × 10@	1 × 12@
AIS Rope Adductors	1 × 8@	1 × 10@	1 × 12@
AIS Rope or Static Quad/Hip	1 × 8@	1 × 10@	1 × 12@
AIS Shoulder (Side-Lying)	1 × 8@	1 × 10@	1 × 12@
AIS Rope Triceps	1 × 8@	1 × 10@	1 × 12@
AIS 90/90 Stretch	1 × 8@	1 × 10@	1 × 12@
AIS Quadruped Rocking	1 × 8	1 × 10	1 × 12

If you're pressed for time, select the 4 AIS stretches that best target your problem areas.

THE CORE WORKOUT

Phase 4: Mixed (Weeks 10, 11, and 12—Week 13 Reload!)
Goals: Speed, Power, Strength, Quality

MONDAY	TUESDAY	WEDNESDAY
Movement Prep A (6 min.)	Movement Prep B (6 min.)	ESD 3 (30 min.)
Elasticity A (10 min.)	Elasticity B (10 min.)	Prehab: Core (5 min.)
Prehab: Shoulder (5 min.)	Strength B (30 min.)	Regeneration: Foam (8 min.)
Strength A (25 min.)	ESD 11 (15 min.)	Regeneration: AIS (10 min.)
ESD 10 (11 min.)	**Total Time: 61 min.**	**Total Time: 53 min.**
Total Time: 57 min.		

STRENGTH: 30-Second Rest between Supersets TEMPO: 30X (Explosive)

STRENGTH A		Monday	Thursday	Monday	Thursday	Monday	Thursday
SUPERSET							
Bench Press+PB Pushup	set 1	6+5	8+5	6+5	8+5	6+5	8+5
	set 2	4+5	6+5	4+5	6+5	4+5	6+5
	set 3	2+5	4+5	2+5	4+5	2+5	4+5
Split Squat+Split Jump	set 1	6+3	8+3	6+3	8+3	6+3	8+3
	set 2	4+3	6+3	4+3	6+3	4+3	6+3
	set 3	2+3	4+3	2+3	4+3	2+3	4+3
SUPERSET							
Kneeling/Cable Lifting	set 1	6@	8@	5@	7@	4@	6@
	set 2	6@	8@	5@	7@	4@	6@
Front Squat-to-Press	set 1	6	8	5	7	4	6
	set 2	6	8	5	7	4	6
DB Pullover Extension	set 1	10	10	8	8	6	6
	set 2	10	10	8	8	6	6

<table>
<tr><td>

THURSDAY
Movement Prep A (6 min.)
Elasticity A (10 min.)
Prehab: Shoulder (5 min.)
Strength A (25 min.)
ESD 10 (11 min.)
Total Time: 57 min.

</td><td>

FRIDAY
Movement Prep B (6 min.)
Elasticity B (10 min.)
Strength B (30 min.)
ESD 11 (15 min.)
Total Time: 61 min.

</td><td>

SATURDAY
ESD 3 (30 min.)
Prehab: Core (5 min.)
Regeneration: Foam (8 min.)
Regeneration: AIS (10 min.)
Total Time: 53 min.

</td></tr>
</table>

Full Range of Motion and Adhere to 30X Tempo!

STRENGTH B		Tuesday	Friday	Tuesday	Friday	Tuesday	Friday
SUPERSET							
Cable 1-Arm Rot. Row	set 1	8@	8@	6@	6@	6@	6@
	set 2	8@	8@	6@	6@	6@	6@
PB Russian Twist	set 1	12	12	15	15	18	18
	set 2	12	12	15	15	18	18
SUPERSET							
1-Arm, 1-Leg DB Row	set 1	6@	8@	5@	7@	4@	6@
	set 2	6@	8@	5@	7@	4@	6@
PB Prone Knee Tuck (1 leg)	set 1	8@	8@	10@	10@	12@	12@
	set 2	8@	8@	10@	10@	12@	12@
SUPERSET							
Romanian Deadlift (1 leg)	set 1	6	6	8	8	10	10
	set 2	6	6	8	8	10	10
PB Reverse Crunch	set 1	12	12	15	15	18	18
	set 2	12	12	15	15	18	18
SUPERSET							
Cable Chopping	set 1	8	8	6	6	4	4
	set 2	8	8	6	6	4	4
DB Curl-to-Press	set 1	6	6	5	5	4	4
	set 2	6	6	5	5	4	4

THE CORE WORKOUT (CONT.)

Phase 4: Mixed (Weeks 10, 11, and 12—Week 13 Reload!)
Goals: Speed, Power, Strength, Quality

MOVEMENT PREP

MOVEMENT PREP A	Week 1	Week 2	Week 3
Forward Lunge/Forearm-to-Instep	1 × 5@	1 × 6@	1 × 7@
Backward Lunge with a Twist	1 × 5@	1 × 6@	1 × 7@
Calf Stretch	1 × 10@	1 × 12@	1 × 7@
Hand Walk	1 × 5	1 × 6	1 × 7
Inverted Hamstring	1 × 5@	1 × 6@	1 × 14@

MOVEMENT PREP B	Week 1	Week 2	Week 3
Hip Crossover	1 × 10@ to 90° knees	1 × 12@ to longer legs	1 × 7@ to straight legs
Scorpion	1 × 10@	1 × 12@	1 × 7@
Lateral Lunge	1 × 5@	1 × 6@	1 × 7@
Drop Lunge	1 × 5@	1 × 6@	1 × 7@
Sumo Squat-to-Stand	1 × 5	1 × 6	1 × 7
Prehab Hip: Glute Bridge (1 leg)	1 × 10@	1 × 12@	1 × 14@

PREHAB

PREHAB: SHOULDER	Week 1	Week 2	Week 3
PB *Y*	1 × 10 + 1 weight	1 × 12 + 1 weight	1 × 12 + 1 weight
PB *T*	1 × 10 + 1 weight	1 × 12 + 1 weight	1 × 12 + 1 weight
PB *W*	1 × 10 + 1 weight	1 × 12 + 1 weight	1 × 12 + 1 weight
PB *L*	1 × 10 + 1 weight	1 × 12 + 1 weight	1 × 12 + 1 weight

PREHAB: CORE	Week 1	Week 2	Week 3
Pillar Bridge Front/Opp Arm/Leg	2–3 × 20 sec.	2–3 × 30 sec.	2–3 × 40 sec.
Pillar Bridge Side (right/left) w/Abduction	2–3 × 20 sec.	2–3 × 30 sec.	2–3 × 40 sec.
Pillar Bridge Side (right/left) w/Adduction	2–3 × 20 sec.	2–3 × 30 sec.	2–3 × 40 sec.

ELASTICITY

ELASTICITY A	Week 1	Week 2	Week 3
Reactive Stepup	2 × 5@	2 × 6@	2 × 6@
Side-to-Side Jump-to-Sprint	4 × 6 jumps each side	4 × 5 jumps each side	4 × 6 jumps each side

ELASTICITY B	Week 1	Week 2	Week 3
Lateral Bound	2 × 6@	2 × 7@	2 × 8@
3-Hurdle Drill	3 × 8 sec.	4 × 8 sec.	4 × 10 sec.

ESD

Workout	Total/# Reps	Warmup	Work/Zone	Rest/Zone
10 Lactate Mixed	11 min./10 reps	3 min./Z1	15 sec./Z3	30 sec./Z1
11 Lactate Mixed	15 min./4 reps	3 min./Z1	1½ min./Z3	1½ min./Z1
3 Aerobic/Recovery	—	—	30+ min./Z1	—

REGENERATION (Done Anytime/Anywhere!)

Exercise	Week 1	Week 2	Week 3
Foam Hamstring	1 × 8@	1 × 10@	1 × 12@
Foam IT Band	1 × 8@	1 × 10@	1 × 12@
Foam Quad/Groin	1 × 8@	1 × 10@	1 × 12@
Foam Glute	1 × 8	1 × 10	1 × 12
Foam Back/Lat	1 × 8@	1 × 10@	1 × 12@
AIS Rope Calf	1 × 8@	1 × 10@	1 × 12@
AIS Rope Hamstring	1 × 8@	1 × 10@	1 × 12@
AIS Rope or Static IT/Glute	1 × 8@	1 × 10@	1 × 12@
AIS Rope Adductors	1 × 8@	1 × 10@	1 × 12@
AIS Rope or Static Quad/Hip	1 × 8@	1 × 10@	1 × 12@
AIS Shoulder (Side-Lying)	1 × 8@	1 × 10@	1 × 12@
AIS Rope Triceps	1 × 8@	1 × 10@	1 × 12@
AIS 90/90 Stretch	1 × 8@	1 × 10@	1 × 12@
AIS Quadruped Rocking	1 × 8	1 × 10	1 × 12

If you're pressed for time, select the 4 AIS stretches that best target your problem areas.

THE CORE WORKOUT
At Home or on the Road

TIME	VERY SHORT		TIME	HAVE A FEW MIN.	
	* Put towel down on floor				
	Extra towel folded up for exercise				
	Clear an alley in the room				
5 Min.	MOVEMENT PREP (MOBILITY)		7 Min.	MOVEMENT PREP (MOBILITY)	
	Hip Crossover	3@		Hip Crossover	5@
	Hand Walk	3		Hand Walk	5
	Forward Lunge/Forearm-to-Instep	3@		Forward Lunge/Forearm-to-Instep	5@
	Backward Lunge with a Twist	3@		Backward Lunge with a Twist	5@
	Lateral Lunge	3@		Lateral Lunge	5@
	Drop Lunge	3@		Drop Lunge	5@
5 Min.	PREHAB		5–10 Min.	PREHAB	
	Shoulder: Floor/PB *Y,T,W,L*	1–2 × 8–15	.	Shoulder: Floor/PB *Y,T,W,L*	1–2 × 8–15
	Hip: Glute Bridge	1–2 × 8–15		Hip: Glute Bridge	1–2 × 8–15
	Core: Pillar Bridge Front	1–2 × 8–15		Core: Pillar Bridge Front	1–2 × 8–15
	Pillar Bridge Side (right/left)	1–2 × 8–15@		Pillar Bridge Side (right/left)	1–2 × 8–15@
5 Min.	ELASTICITY		7–12 Min.	ELASTICITY	
	Base Side-to-Side	1–2 × 5–10 sec.		Base Side-to-Side	1–2 × 5–10 sec.
	Base Rotation	1–2 × 5–10 sec.		Base Rotation	1–2 × 5–10 sec.
	1 Leg over the Line	1–2 × 5–10 sec.		1 Leg over the Line	1–2 × 5–10 sec.
	Squat Jump	1–3 × 4–6		Split Jump	1–3 × 3–4
	Plyo Pushup	1–3 × 4–6		Reactive Stepup (Stairwell)	1–3 × 4–6@
				Plyo Pushup	1–3 × 4–6
5 Min.	STRENGTH		10 Min.	STRENGTH	
	Floor/PB Pushup Plus	1–3 × 8–30+		Floor/PB Pushup Plus	1–3 × 4–30
	Split Squat/Lunge	1–3 × 8–30+@		Floor/PB Leg Curl	1–3 × 4–12
				Split Squat/Lunge	1–3 × 4–15@
0 Min.	ESD		6–20 Min.	ESD	
	Take the stairs and walk today			Stairs: Every 2–3 Stairs	
	Eat great . . . be disciplined			# of Flights	Beginner: 10
					Intermediate: 15
					Advanced: 20+
				*Take Elevator Down to Repeat	
0 Min.	REGENERATION		0 Min.	REGENERATION	
	Evening if Option			Evening if Option	
	Rope			Rope	
	Water: Shower/Bath/Pool			Water: Shower/Bath/Pool	

*NOTE: Create some time for your A.M. workout by electing for a preworkout shooter/snack and postworkout shake!

**DB curl then front squat-to-press: We will be combining 2 exercises here. Do a heavy DB curl, then go into your front squat-to-press, lower weights to the shoulders, then lower the DB down to your hips, and repeat w/ DB curl.

TIME	FULL WITH HOME/HOTEL WT. ROOM	
7 Min.	MOVEMENT PREP (MOBILITY)	
	Hip Crossover	5@
	Hand Walk	5
	Forward Lunge/Forearm-to-Instep	5@
	Backward Lunge with a Twist	5@
	Lateral Lunge	5@
	Drop Lunge	5@
5–10 Min.	PREHAB	
	Shoulder: Floor/PB Y,T,W,L	1 × 8–15
	Hip: Glute Bridge	1 × 8–15
	Core: Pillar Bridge Front	1 × 8–15
	Pillar Bridge Side (right/left)	1 × 8–15@
7–12 Min.	ELASTICITY	
	Base Side-to-Side	1–2 × 5–10 sec.
	Base Rotation	1–2 × 5–10 sec.
	1 Leg Over the Line	1–2 × 5–10 sec.
	Split Jump	1–3 × 3–4
	Reactive Stepup	1–3 × 4–6@
	Plyo Pushup	1 × 3–10
10–25 Min.	STRENGTH CIRCUIT #1	
	Bench Press (Bar or DB)	1–3 × 4–15
	1-Arm, 1-Leg DB Row	1–3 × 4–15@
	Split Squat/Lunge	1–3 × 4–15@
	Romanian Deadlift	1–3 × 4–15
	DB Pullover Extension	1–3 × 4–15
	DB Curl Front Squat-to-Press	1–3 × 4–15
	OR	
	10-MIN. STRENGTH BLAST	
	DB Curl then Front Squat-to-Press**	1–3 × 6–15
	Romanian Deadlift (DB)	1–3 × 6–15
	ESD (Your Choice between Level 4–9)	
	Incline Intervals on Treadmill/Bike	10–20 min.
	OR	
	Run Stairs	
	Singles, Doubles, or Triples	10–20 min.
	Walk back down to start laterally	10–20 min.

PRIOR TO FLIGHT

Movement Prep + Prehab Short
Drink a lot of water hours before the flight
Include antioxidant complex + vitamin C
Get as rested as possible
If sleeping flight, have a higher carbohydrate meal
  rich in antioxidants before getting on plane and
  hydrate—this will assist you in falling asleep
Set watch to new time zone upon entering plane

DURING THE FLIGHT

Drink 4 ounces every 15 minutes
Upon arrival Movement Prep, Prehab AIS Stretch
Make sure to continue to wash hands
Get up and stretch hip flexors/hamstring/lats,
  adductors/chest in galley area
Self-massage
Bring your own food—don't forget those meal-
  replacement bars, jerky, nuts, or fruit
Bring your shaker bottle and vitamins
Move the pillow in and out of lumbar spine

AFTER THE FLIGHT

If sleeping flight, wake up on new time zone
Hydrate, antioxidant complex
Higher protein meal (stimulate your mind)
Get into the sun to adjust body clock
Wash hands and keep away from face
Movement Prep, Prehab Short, AIS Stretch

TRAVELING WITH SUPPLEMENTS

Zip-top snack bags (for fiber, glutamine, etc.)
Mix fiber in with protein
Put vitamins in snack bags
Put above and plastic spoon in shaker bottle
Don't forget to put some goodies in briefcase and bag
  (meal-replacement bars, jerky, nuts, water)
Toothbrush and hand wipes will help protect the immune
  system

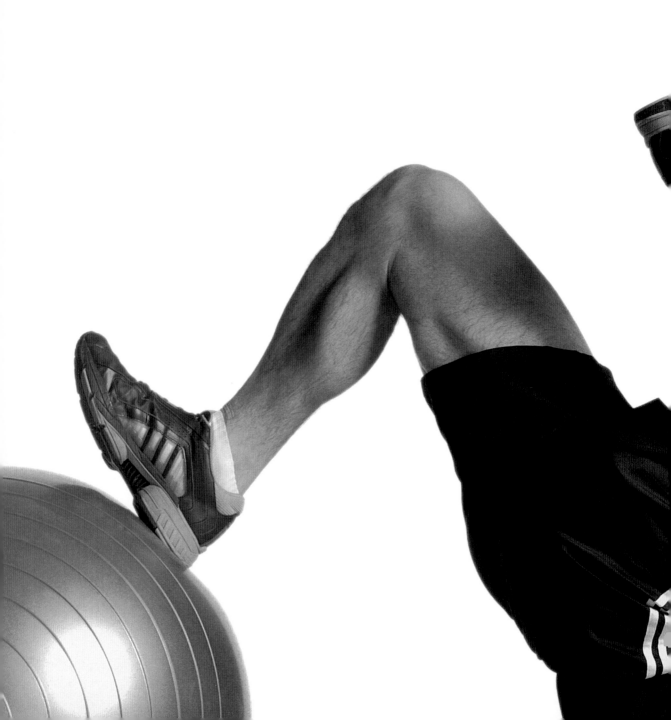

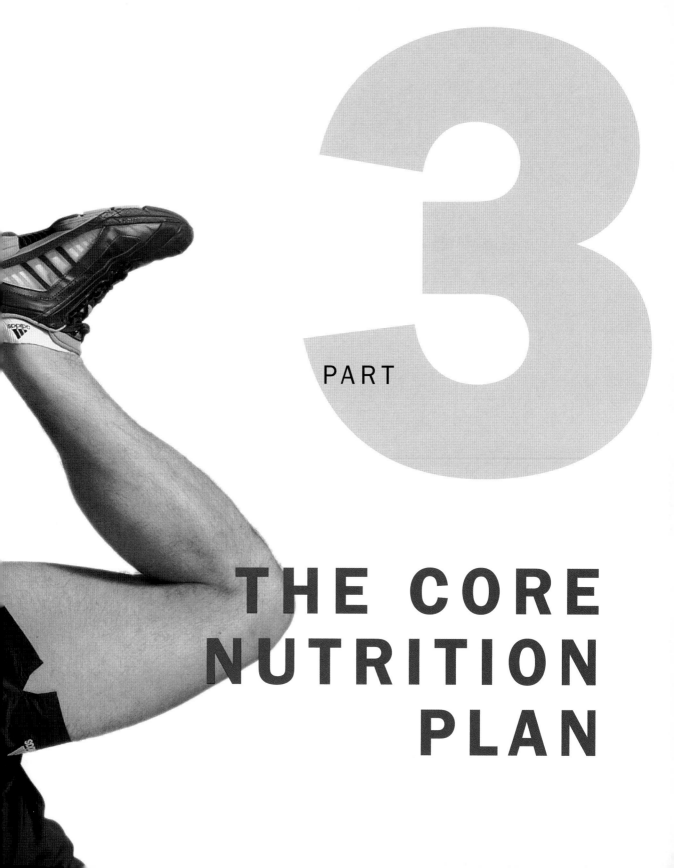

PART

3

THE CORE
NUTRITION
PLAN

CHAPTER 13

HOW TO EAT BETTER, STARTING NOW

Like most people, you've probably been on a diet at some point in your life. Maybe you've followed one of the most recent fads, counting your calories or focusing on your intake of carbohydrates, fats, and proteins. You've no doubt heard countless ads for miracle supplements that supposedly help you lose weight or gain energy.

All of those strategies tend to address the symptoms—too much weight and lack of energy—rather than the problem, which is a poor nutrition program. The Core Nutrition Plan is a way to maximize energy, lose fat, gain lean mass, and save money and time.

You're going to have five or six meals and snacks a day, which means you get to eat something every 2½ to 3 hours. If you eat often, your body becomes a more efficient energy-burning machine. Not only that, frequent eating keeps you from overeating. If you know you're going to have something in a few hours, you'll be less likely to overeat—and less likely to be extremely hungry.

The reason most people don't eat well is because they don't plan ahead, so they end up devouring whatever they can grab. The process of stressing out over where and when to eat is unhealthy, a problem made worse by the junk you inevitably consume in such a state. As a result, you end up increasing body fat and decreasing lean mass, which defeats the purpose of following the Core Workout. Not only that, but eating on the run is expensive. It costs more, and it takes a toll on your health.

Like everything else in this book, I want you to be proactive about your diet. My wife and I spend 90 minutes each Sunday planning, shopping, and preparing menus of meals for an entire week. It's easy and fun—and it saves money. In chapter 14, I'll give you a shopping list of acceptable foods, then guide you through the grocery store and back to your kitchen to lay out healthy, delicious meals for the entire week. You'll save time and money and won't need to stress out about meals.

Eating well, like working out properly, is a matter of understanding a few concepts and then planning to implement them. And if you have the proper nutrition system in place, you'll find that eating healthy is less stressful, less expensive, and more enjoyable.

I'll show you how to get the most nutrients out of your foods and how to create a championship meal plan with the proper intakes of proteins, carbs, fats, fiber, vitamins, and minerals. You'll see how to combine foods for a powerful nutritional value and to maximize energy. As with the Core Workout, you want to get the best return on the investment you make in your meals.

Entire books have been written about carbs or proteins alone. Let's keep it simple. I'll cut through the hype and the fad diets to show you what is supported by science. Here are 10 coaching keys that will give you everything you need to know about nutrition.

COACHING KEY NO. 1: EAT SMALLER AMOUNTS MORE OFTEN

Our culture promotes the idea of getting three square meals a day, avoiding between-meal snacks, and not eating between dinner and bedtime. Is it any wonder that we tend to feel bloated from overeating those three square meals, hungry and lethargic during the long periods between meals, and starved before bedtime?

Forget what you've been taught. If you want to control your appetite, regulate your blood sugar level to stay energized and alert, and build lean body mass, you must eat five or six small- to medium-size meals or snacks each day. That means you need to eat, on average, every 3 hours. Think of yourself as "grazing" all day, instead of sitting down for three massive feedings.

Controlling blood sugar levels improves concentration and helps regulate appetite. If you can do those two things, you'll be in much better control of your body. After all, having consistent levels of blood sugar gives you consistent energy and makes you feel good, since you're avoiding huge swings in hunger and mood.

Over the course of the day, your mood, concentration, and energy levels go up and down. Aside from the stresses of your day, this is partly a function of your blood sugar levels. When these levels go down, there's a tendency to grab the first food available, and that's usually not something good for you.

Frequent eating is like constantly throwing wood on the fire. Digesting food cranks up your metabolism and burns more calories every time you eat. By not eating often, the fire smolders and dies. A hot fire, on the other hand, burns wood continuously. Those six smaller meals keep the fire hot. And since you know you'll eat in a few hours, you're less likely to overeat.

It's possible to fit in six meals a day regardless of your job or lifestyle. Remember that our six "meals" are not going to be long, sit-down affairs. A few could be, but three of those meals are going to be snacks; one or two of those will be preworkout "shooters"—juice or water mixed with some whey protein—or post-workout recovery shakes. And since you're eating more often, your traditional breakfasts, lunches, and dinners probably will be lighter.

If we don't eat often, the most readily available substance for the body to consume is muscle. There's a misconception that the body first eats away its fat. But the body is remarkably resistant to fat loss and will turn to its lean muscle first, keeping that stored body fat in reserve as long as necessary.

Remember Pac-Man and Ms. Pac-Man from those 1980s video games? They needed to eat constantly to keep going. Think of your body as Mr. and Ms. Pac-Man, constantly looking for fuel. If they can't find any, they'll get irritable, like a dog that needs to be fed. If the dog can't find food, he'll chew on the couch or a pillow. Mr. and Ms. Pac-Man chomp on your lean muscle.

Many people try to get thin by not eating. They deprive their bodies of nutrients and, while they might look healthy, they have dangerous blood profiles and a high ratio of fat to lean muscle. Their bodies are what I call "skinny fat."

The last thing we want to do is lose lean mass. After all, we've put forth a tremendous effort through the Core Workout to build this lean mass, which produces power, stabilizes joints, promotes movement, and is critical for optimal performance throughout life, not to mention on the athletic field. We lose a pound of lean mass per year as we age, so it's imperative to take action to maintain this lean mass.

To do that, we must eat often, which brings us to our next coaching key. . . .

COACHING KEY NO. 2: TIMING IS EVERYTHING

You might think there's no way you can fit in six meals a day, given your busy schedule. But if you plan it out, you'll save the time spent wondering what you're going to eat. And since you'll have your meals planned, you'll be less likely to be in that starving state that usually results in eating the first thing available.

Here are three ways to schedule your six meals, depending on whether you work out in the morning, over lunch, or after work. I've also included some menu suggestions and a schedule for those who compete in early evening sporting events.

Option A: For Those Who Work Out Before Work or School

6:15 A.M.:	Preworkout shooter
6:30–7:30 A.M.:	**Workout**
7:30 A.M.:	Meal #1 (**Breakfast:** Egg-white omelet with vegetables; fruit and oatmeal)
10:30 A.M.:	Meal #2 (Shake or Snack)
1:30 P.M.:	Meal #3 (**Lunch:** Tuna with fat-free mayonnaise and/or celery, lettuce, and tomato on rye bread, or as a salad)
4:00–4:30 P.M.:	Meal #4 (Shake or Snack)
7:00–7:30 P.M.:	Meal #5 (**Dinner:** Grilled salmon with vegetables and couscous)
10:00–10:30 P.M.:	Meal #6 (Shake or Snack)

Option B: For Those Who Work Out during Lunch Hour

7:00 A.M.:	Meal #1 (**Breakfast:** Oatmeal and a *small* piece of deli meat)
10:00 A.M.:	Meal #2 (Shake or Snack)
11:45 A.M.:	Preworkout shooter
Noon–1:00 P.M.:	**Workout**
1:00 P.M.:	Meal #3 (**Lunch:** Chicken breast on sourdough, pumpernickel, or rye bread, with fruit and vegetables)

4:00 P.M.:	Meal #4 (Shake or Snack)
7:00 P.M.:	Meal #5 (**Dinner:** A grilled cut of lean red meat with brown or wild rice and vegetables)
10:00 P.M.:	Meal #6 (Shake or Snack)

Option C: For Those Who Work Out after Work

7:00 A.M.:	Meal #1 (**Breakfast:** A bowl of Kashi cereal with blueberries)
10:00 A.M.:	Meal #2 (Shake or Snack)
1:00 P.M.:	Meal #3 (**Lunch:** Chicken breast on a bed of spinach or lettuce with sliced tomatoes, a small sprinkling of nuts, and olive oil for dressing)
4:00 P.M.:	Meal #4 (Shake or Snack)
5:30–6:30 P.M.:	**Workout**
6:30 P.M.:	Meal #5 (**Dinner:** Lean pork in Shake 'n Bake seasoning with rice and vegetables)
9:30 P.M.:	Meal #6 (Shake or Snack)

Option D: For Those Competing in the Early Evening

7:00 A.M.:	Meal #1 (**Breakfast:** Low-fat, low-sugar yogurt with flaxseed oil and/or oatmeal)
10:00 A.M.:	Meal #2 (Shake or Snack)

1:00 P.M.:	Meal #3 (**Lunch:** Lean turkey on rye, pumpernickel, or sourdough bread, with vegetables or as a salad)
4:00 P.M.:	Meal #4 (Shake or Snack)
6:00 P.M.:	Meal #5 (**Dinner:** Seasoned grilled swordfish fillet with vegetables)
7:00 P.M.:	**Game/Competition**
9:00–9:30 P.M.:	Meal #6 (Postworkout shake or snack with flaxseed oil)

This might seem as if you're eating a lot, but it's not if you consume *smaller* portions. We've become accustomed, especially in the United States, to eating supersize servings. Fast-food restaurants now refer to them as "value" sizes, to make you feel good about getting more for your money, even though you're still pigging out on junk.

One of the best ways to avoid overeating and maintain a healthy metabolism is to pay attention to your portion sizes. By eating smaller portions more often, you give your body a better chance to digest and get all of the nutrients from the food. A good rule of thumb is that a piece of fish or meat should be about the size of a deck of cards, and a serving of starches (rice or pasta, for example) should be no bigger than the size of a fist. You can eat as many vegetables as you like.

Most people eat dinner around 7:00 P.M. and don't eat again until breakfast. That's as much as 12 hours without food—even longer if you skip breakfast. Your body gets through this extended fast by tapping into your lean muscle for nourishment. That's why I want to shrink that noneating window to 8 to 10 hours. (If you have that last snack at 10:00 P.M. and breakfast at 6:00 A.M., you can minimize the fast while getting a full night's sleep.) We'll talk more about appropriate snacks later in this chapter.

You never want your body to be in a fasted state, especially when you work out. Yet many people exercise first thing in the morning on an empty stomach. Don't get me wrong; exercising is a great way to start the day. In fact, that's my only time to work out. But eat something before your workout, even if it's just half an apple or a preworkout shooter. That can be a very watered-down glass of orange juice with a scoop of whey protein, a glass of water with the scoop of whey, or green tea with a low-carbohydrate meal-replacement bar. Perhaps the best convenient grab-and-go solution is EAS Myoplex Lite, which has 25 grams of protein, 20 grams of carbs, 5 grams of fiber, and 2.5 grams of fat. You can find it at many supermarkets and health food stores.

Whey gets into your system quickly, which is especially important if you're eating prior to or immediately following a workout. You'll note that you can consume as many as three

WHEY TO GO ■

Try to take at least one serving a day of whey protein. Whey (pronounced "way") is a by-product of cheese manufacturing and includes many essential amino acids that boost the immune system and promote overall good health.

You'll get whey protein in postworkout recovery mixes like the ones you'll use in this program, but you might want to try one additional serving. It's available in powdered form in a number of flavors and tastes great sprinkled on oatmeal or mixed with milk, water, or juice.

protein-rich shakes a day under this plan, but you're not required to drink three. (Recommended brands include Myoplex Deluxe Low-Carb by EAS; General Nutrition Center's Mega MRP, which is part of its Pro Performance Elite series; and the Total Nutrition drink mix manufactured by Met-Rx.)

The value of these shakes is that they accelerate workout recovery, build lean body mass, and account for 40 to 100 percent of the daily recommended allowance of 25 vitamins and minerals per serving. Since the shakes can be made by mixing water with a scoop or packet of powder in a covered plastic container or blender, they're a quick, easy, and portable snack that won't spoil.

Some people find it challenging to consume three shakes a day. They quickly grow tired of them. I can appreciate that, which is why I require you to have only one shake a day—either immediately before or after your workout.

Ideally, you should have a shake right after the workout. At that point, your cells are wide open and screaming for nutrients. By having a shake immediately after working out, you're expediting the recovery process and maximizing lean-muscle growth.

That said, most people like to exercise first thing in the morning, during lunch, or after work. So it might be more convenient for you to follow a meal schedule like the one we discussed earlier and consume a shooter before working out. Recent research has shown that a whey protein shooter may give you an effect equal or superior to a traditional postworkout recovery shake. The preworkout shooter works its way into the bloodstream to give the muscle exactly what it needs at the earliest possible moment. It's like giving your muscles a flying start toward recovery. Athletes in training will benefit most from a preworkout carbohydrate-protein source. If weight control is a concern, however, focus on the protein and minimize carbs in the preworkout shooter.

Some other recent research shows that if you've had that preworkout shooter, it's okay to wait 45 minutes to an hour after working out before eating. The research suggests that the wait will help you burn calories and lose weight.

You might consider adding a teaspoon of each of three powerful amino acids to your pre-workout shooter or postworkout recovery shake: Glutamine supports the body's immune and digestive systems. Taurine assists in the digestion of fats. And leucine helps build lean body mass.

That final snack or shake at 10:00 P.M. should include something high in protein, since that helps build lean muscle. You also want fiber and essential fats (such as fish or flaxseed oil). For many people, a protein shake or high-protein meal-replacement bar might be an easy option. A piece of fruit is a good choice as well, since it's full of antioxidants and jump-starts the regenerative process. So an ideal bedtime snack could be a protein shake with a teaspoon of flaxseed oil and a handful of blue-berries.

Because everyone who reads this will be on a slightly different schedule, there's no one-size-fits-all routine I can offer. But if you re-member the priorities—eating often and getting either a preworkout shooter or a postworkout recovery shake in—you can plan your day ac-cordingly.

My wife and I find that the easiest way to plan our meals is to do our shopping for the week on Sunday, making up as many conve-nient and tasty meals as possible and sticking them in the refrigerator.

This preparation doesn't account for all of our meals, but it provides a good starting point for eating right over the course of the week. It covers the majority of our lunches and provides a few nutritious, ready-to-eat dinners for those nights when we get home late.

One way to get a lot of your meal planning out of the way is to grill plenty of chicken, fish, and *lean* red meat on Sunday and place it in one-serving plastic containers that have sepa-rate compartments. Place some salad and veg-etables in the other compartments, and you're set for lunch. When you come home, dinner is ready, since all you have to do, at most, is steam some vegetables.

Planning this way also helps save money, since you're less likely to end up in that hur-ried, fasted state in which the blood sugar is so low that you're willing to eat anything you can find, no matter how bad it is for you. Too often, what you find is a restaurant of one kind or another—expensive, takeout, fast-food—and after a while those meals add up.

Speaking of Sundays, since it's an "off" day from the Core Workout, feel free to take the day off nutritionally as well. This doesn't mean that you should inhale an entire pizza with a six-pack of beer and an apple pie, but it's okay to treat yourself. You've worked hard the entire week and deserve to relax. Not only that, but having that treat provides a psycho-logical benefit: It helps you realize that you're not completely depriving yourself of foods you enjoy, even if they aren't particularly good for you. Physiologically, it helps present a depressed metabolism if you're trying to lose weight by reducing your daily calorie intake.

It's unrealistic to think that you're going to eat nothing but healthy foods 42 times a week (six meals a day for 7 days). So take Sundays off. Remember, even pros who train at Athletes' Performance—a group that includes some of the most disciplined, dedicated people you'll ever meet—allow themselves an occasional indulgence.

When planning meals, it's vital to consider the role of carbohydrates, proteins, and fats. Contrary to popular belief, they must all be included in a nutrition plan for optimal performance.

Carbs are our fuel, though the amount of carbs we eat must be proportional to our activity level. If I fill up my car's gas tank, drive 5 miles, and then try to fill it up again, it's going to overflow. Unlike your car, you might not realize you're overfilling your tank and contributing to a higher level of body fat.

Generally speaking, the higher the activity level, the more carbs you want to consume. Since most people tend to be more active in the morning and afternoon, it makes sense to eat the majority of your carbs earlier in the day. Your body's glucose tolerance—its ability to metabolize carbohydrates and push them into muscles for energy—is also strongest at these times.

Every meal should include fruits and vegetables because of their fiber and nutrient densities. I recommend that you "eat a rainbow often," which refers not only to the bright colors of fruits and vegetables but also to the need to eat six small meals and snacks a day. Typically, your plate should consist mostly of colorful, high-fiber vegetables. There should be a piece of meat or fish the size of a deck of cards and, if you like, a fist-size (or smaller) portion of rice or pasta. There also should be some "good" fats in the form of, say, salmon or olive oil. (We'll discuss fats in more detail later in this chapter.)

COACHING KEY NO. 3: ALL CARBS ARE NOT CREATED EQUAL

The glycemic index is a useful tool to measure how quickly a single food will raise your blood glucose level. To illustrate, let's compare broccoli to cotton candy. If you eat 100 calories of cotton candy, it dissolves quickly in your mouth and is absorbed immediately, sending your blood sugar level sky-high. Give kids a high-glycemic food like cotton candy, and they'll bounce off the walls. Even adults feel a sugar rush.

The problem is that you crash quickly and end up feeling sluggish. Your body then craves more sugar. Cotton candy, not surprisingly, has a very high glycemic-index number.

"THE DEVIL'S CARB" ■

In the 1980s, low-fat and nonfat diets became a national obsession. With everyone looking to avoid fat, food manufacturers took all the fat out of their products. But since they still wanted the food to taste good, they dumped additional high-fructose corn syrup into it to make up for the good taste the fat provided.

The reduced fat and added sugar made the foods higher on the glycemic index, sending our blood sugar levels sky-high before crashing quickly, making our bodies hungry for more high-glycemic food.

As a result, people got into that vicious cycle of eating more and more high-glycemic food to maintain that blood sugar rush, rather than eating foods the body needs to control appetite and blood sugar level.

According to a study published in *The American Journal of Clinical Nutrition,* Americans ate an average of about a half a pound of high-fructose corn syrup in 1970. By 1997, we were consuming up to 62½ pounds each!

Unfortunately, this sweetener is in everything, from soft drinks to barbecue sauce and ketchup to canned soups and juices. Is it any wonder that obesity rates have soared over the last three decades?

There's nothing wrong with a little high-fructose corn syrup, but when you look at a label, see how prominent it is. If it's listed first or second in the ingredients list, glance at the product's nutrition-facts label to see how much sugar is in the product. If it's more than 8 grams per serving, find a different brand or, if necessary, a healthier substitute. Generally speaking, avoid products with high-fructose corn syrup.

If you eat 100 calories of broccoli, however, it takes your body much longer to break it down and release the blood sugar. You have to chew it—really chew it, if it's cooked so it retains some crunch—and your mouth releases digestive enzymes to help. Think of Pac-Man and Ms. Pac-Man gradually chomping that broccoli in your tummy. It's going to take them more time. But there's a nice benefit to all that slow chomping. Sugar from the food will be released into your bloodstream over a longer period, and the soluble fiber that broccoli provides slowing gastrointestinal transit. Broccoli, therefore, has a low glycemic-index number.

We want to eat mostly lower to moderately rated glycemic foods (the one exception is right after a workout). But since we rarely eat just one food at a time, we need to think about the body's overall glycemic *response* to everything on our plate. If we have a high-glycemic food with some low-glycemic foods, the overall glycemic response is moderate, which is fine.

Another way to think of this is in terms of the glycemic *load,* which is computed by taking the food's glycemic index and multiplying by .01, then multiplying that total by the number of calories per serving. I don't expect you to actually do this, but the thing to remember is that the larger the portion of a high-glycemic carb, the higher the glycemic load will be.

For instance, orange juice is highly glycemic. It will send your blood sugar level soaring. A smaller glass obviously will have a smaller glycemic load than a larger serving. You also could lower the glycemic response of the orange juice by diluting it further with water.

Your body's glycemic response is often individual—your response to a food probably won't be exactly the same as mine. The important thing is for you to recognize how different foods will affect your blood sugar levels and to take note of any that have a particular effect on you.

Generally speaking, the lower the number on the glycemic index, the less processed the food will be. Your body has to do the work to get the nutrients out of these foods, and that's good because that gradual release helps regulate blood sugar levels. Look for natural foods that have more color and fiber, since they control appetite, have more nutrients, and improve the health of your cardiovascular system. (I emphasize the word *natural* since, after all, cotton candy can be found in a lot of colors.)

By controlling your blood sugar, you're regulating the hormone insulin. If you're constantly jacking up your blood sugar level by eating only high-glycemic foods, crashing back down, and then eating more high-glycemic foods, you create a vicious cycle that results in increased body-fat levels, followed by obesity and perhaps even diabetes.

The reason we see so many overweight children these days, aside from an utter lack of exercise, is that the majority of things we feed them are highly processed, high-sugar, high-glycemic foods that wreak havoc on blood sugar levels and provide little nutritional value. Not only does this have serious health implications, but a kid eating poorly could have attention deficits and wild mood swings that will affect development and performance.

Examples of low- or slow-glycemic foods include sweet potatoes, yams, green peas, black beans, oatmeal (not instant), peaches, oranges, apples, grapefruit, cherries, and fat-free milk. Moderate-glycemic foods include mashed potatoes, sweet corn, bananas, cantaloupe, pineapple, whole grain bread, cheese pizza, and oatmeal cookies. High-glycemic foods include baked potatoes, doughnuts, waffles, bagels, raisin bran, graham crackers, pretzels, corn chips, watermelon, juices, and sweetened breakfast cereals made from refined grains.

If you find that a food produces an unexpected result, either high or low, take note of it and incorporate it into your meal planning. For example, you can balance the effect of a high-glycemic carbohydrate food by combining it with a low-glycemic carbohydrate and/or protein and "good" fats. The result is to produce a meal that, on balance, is a moderate carb. The way a food is prepared also can impact its glycemic rating. If pasta is slightly undercooked, it has a lower value on the glycemic

A WORD ON FIBER ■

Try to consume a lot of fiber. Fiber improves your body's digestive function, regulates blood sugar levels, and promotes long-term cardiovascular health. It's found in oatmeal and green, leafy vegetables as well as in bottled form. You can sprinkle it on your meals to improve their nutritional value. Because fiber is found mostly in carbohydrates and is essential to overall health, people who follow low-carb diet plans are depriving themselves of this vital source of nutrition.

---

index. The less prepared a carbohydrate is, the better it is for you.

The important thing to remember is that carbs are not inherently bad, as the authors of several popular diet plans would lead you to believe. Carbs that are highly processed and low in fiber and that include high-fructose corn syrup (or HFCS) are the ones to avoid.

Admittedly, not eating carbs is one way to lose a lot of weight in a hurry. After all, for every gram of carbohydrate we eat, we store 3 grams of water. But that's not so bad. Water keeps us hydrated and satiated.

If you go on one of those diets without carbs, it's like taking a sponge and wringing the water out. You'll lose the water weight, but as soon as you eat carbs again—and you will at some point because you need energy and can only go so long without carbs—then that sponge is going to fill up with water. When it does, the weight comes right back. Plus, you'll likely lose some of your lean mass.

Too many carbs is a bad thing only if your activity level is low or you're consuming a lot of high-glycemic carbs with little nutritional value.

Overall, carbs are an important part of your diet when you consume them relative to your activity level and within the context of the glycemic index.

COACHING KEY NO. 4: KNOW YOUR PROTEINS

Protein is critical to have with every meal because it builds and maintains muscles. It's responsible for healthy blood cells and key enzymes, and it strengthens the immune system, which fights off infection and disease.

Yet, protein will only be used to build muscle if you eat enough carbohydrate calories to provide the body with energy. Otherwise, your body will tap into the protein for energy.

I recommend that you consume between 0.6 and 0.8 gram of protein per pound of body weight. If you weigh, say, 180 pounds, you would want to shoot for between 108 and 144 grams of protein per day. Generally speaking, the leaner you are and the higher your activity level, the higher your protein intake should be on that scale.

That might sound like a ton of protein—and it is a significant amount—but consider how much protein is in common foods such as the ones listed below.

Chicken (4 ounces, skinless): 35 grams
Tuna (6 ounces, packed in water):
  40 grams
Fish (6 ounces of cod or salmon):
  40 grams
Lean pork (4 ounces): 35 grams
Low-fat tofu (6 ounces): 30 grams
Cottage cheese (1 cup of 1% or 2% fat):
  28 grams
Lean red meat (4 ounces): 35 grams
Milk (1 cup of low-fat or fat-free): 8 grams

Remember, too, that your preworkout shooter or postworkout recovery mix is going to contain 20 to 45 grams of protein per serving. If you have one or two shakes a day, along with some combination of poultry and fish for lunch and dinner and a breakfast that includes yogurt or egg whites, you'll easily meet your daily protein goal.

In addition to "eat a rainbow often," here's another rule of thumb regarding nutrition, specifically protein: "The less legs, the better." My colleague Tracy Morgan came up with this to refer to the fact that the fewer legs something has—or at least had when it was alive—the better its ratio of protein to fat.

Fish, for instance, have no legs, and fish is a tremendously healthy source of protein, provided it's not fried or marinated in fat. Fish also provides omega-3 and omega-6 fatty acids, which promote cardiovascular health. Chickens have two legs and also are a wonderful source of protein, provided the skin is removed and the meat is not fried.

Meat from four-legged creatures can be good, too, provided it's a lean cut of meat. That's a key distinction. Red meat gets a bad rap, some of which is deserved since there's so much fatty meat for sale at supermarkets and restaurants. But lean red meat is a tremendous source of important nutrients such as iron, phosphorus, and creatine.

Pork, the so-called "other white meat," also gets a bad rap. It's usually fatty, but if you ask your butcher for a lean cut with little marbling, you'll have a nutritious protein.

COACHING KEY NO. 5: FATS ARE FABULOUS

One of the biggest health trends of the last 20 years has been the antifat movement. Everything had to be low-fat, preferably fat-free. "You are what you eat," according to the popular saying, and if you ate fat, you were going to end up a fat tub of goo.

Fats are critical to good health. Cell membranes are made of fat. Fats release energy slowly, keeping the body satiated and regulating blood sugar, and thus lowering your

LEGS, RAINBOWS, AND WINE ■

Baseball players Nomar Garciaparra and Lou Merloni have worked with me for nearly a decade and have memorized many of my favorite sayings, such as "eat a rainbow often" and "the less legs, the better." They're always trying to come up with exceptions to my rules, if only for the sake of argument.

One night over dinner, Nomar raised his glass of red wine and said, "You know, wine comes from grapes."

Lou nodded. "It also has good color. Red *is* in the rainbow."

Nomar swirled his glass like the consummate wine connoisseur. "And this wine has good legs."

Better wines are said to have "good legs," in reference to the little rivulets that collect on the inside of a wine glass and indicate overall richness and power of the wine.

"I'd say this wine is an acceptable part of our program," Lou said.

I laughed. I rarely drink wine but had to agree, although technically with wine you would say, "the *more* legs, the better."

Numerous studies have suggested that moderate consumption of red wine reduces the risk of cardio-vascular disease. Resveratrol, an antioxidant, is naturally found in high concentrations in red grape skins. Some wines include juice from other antioxidant-rich fruits such as plums, cherries, and berries. So there is some health benefit to drinking wine.

Now I'm not suggesting that you add wine to your nutrition program. Alcohol should be consumed only in moderation. But if you have an occasional glass of wine, particularly red wine, you can rest assured that it's an acceptable part of the Core Nutrition Plan.

---

glycemic response to the other foods you're eating. Fats help get you from meal to meal without feeling as if you're starving, and they give your body some powerful nutrients and antioxidants for cellular repair of the joints, organs, skin, and hair. Fats, especially those found in fish oil and flaxseed oil, also help with cognitive ability, mental clarity, and memory retention.

Not all fat is good, of course. You want to eat *unsaturated* fats, not saturated. The difference in chemical structure of the two produces significantly different effects on health. Saturated fats raise serum cholesterol levels, clog arteries, and pose a threat to your heart. Unsaturated fats do not raise cholesterol levels, and research indicates they actually reduce blood cholesterol levels when substituted for saturated fats.

Unsaturated fats are liquid at room temperature and are found in foods such as olive oil, canola oil, flaxseed oil, and fish oils.

Not all unsaturated fats are healthy, though. Vegetable shortening is also unsaturated, but when it's used to fry foods, it's unhealthy. That's because it contains trans fats, which raise bad (LDL) cholesterol but do not raise good (HDL) cholesterol. This artery-clogging fat is found in processed foods such as cookies, crackers, pies, pastries, and margarine. It's also found in fried foods, especially those at fast-food restaurants, and in smaller quantities in meat and some dairy products. As of January 1, 2006, food manufacturers must list on their labels the amount of trans fat; some manufacturers have done so already. Even snack foods labeled "low-fat" contain too much trans fat, so be sure to consult the labels.

The best fats come out of nuts, fish oils, and seeds. Few foods have such an undeserved bad rap as nuts. As part of the antifat movement, people avoided nuts since they were high in fat. But nuts and seeds are a good, convenient source of protein, fiber, and positive fats, and they stick with you longer, helping control your blood sugar and appetite. A handful of nuts every day can lower your risk of heart ailments and Alzheimer's disease. You don't want to scarf down an entire can of nuts, but a small serving is a good snack, especially if combined with, say, a glass of fat-free milk. A quarter-cup (about the size of a packet you might get on an airplane) is a good serving size. Nuts also make a nutritious topping for salads and main courses. In a recent rating of nuts by *Men's Health* magazine, almonds were found to have the most nutritional value, followed by cashews, pecans, and macadamias.

The opposite of nuts getting a bad rap would be fat-free yogurt having an undeserved good reputation. Not all yogurts are created equal. Fat-free yogurt often is loaded with empty calories and heavy in sugar, which will send your blood sugar level soaring.

A better bet is low-fat, low-sugar yogurt, which tastes better, sticks with you longer, and helps regulate blood sugar levels. It also can be a good source of protein and digestive enzymes. Add in some extra fiber, nuts, or flaxseeds. It's also tasty when mixed with oatmeal.

Fish oils provide powerful omega-3 and omega-6 fatty acids, which have antioxidant properties and are essential for good cardiovascular health and mental clarity. These are found in salmon, mackerel, lake trout, herring, sardines, and some types of white fish. Swordfish and tuna have fatty acids, though not as much as salmon. Fish is a tremendous source of protein without the high saturated fats found in fatty meat products.

Everyone should have a bottle of flaxseed oil and fish oil in the refrigerator. The body can convert flaxseed oil into omega-3 and omega-6 fatty acids, much like fish oil. A tablespoon or two a day, one in the morning and one in the evening, is all you need, and it can go into a shake or on top of oatmeal.

Olive oil is another excellent choice for

cooking. It has great antioxidant properties, is good for cooking, and goes well with salads.

Now that we've straightened out the common misperceptions about fats (as well as carbs and protein) as individual units, we're ready to talk specifically about combining them to form powerful meals with the best glycemic response and nutritional value. It all starts with the next coaching key.

COACHING KEY NO. 6: BREAKFAST *IS* THE MOST IMPORTANT MEAL OF THE DAY

Think of breakfast as "break-the-fast," which is exactly what you're doing. When you wake up in the morning, your body is in a fasted state. During sleep, it uses the available nutrients for repair and energy, and by the time you wake up, there's usually nothing left. Your tank is empty, and Mr. and Ms. Pac-Man will turn to your lean-muscle stores for energy.

Since we'll have a nutrient-dense, slow-releasing snack before bedtime, we're going to give the body what it wants so it doesn't tap into its lean-muscle stores. Breakfast is going to ensure that your body doesn't consume its muscle for food, a process known as *catabolism.* Breakfast also increases metabolism, fuels the brain, and provides energy.

Too many people substitute caffeine, specifically coffee, to get an artificial energy and metabolism boost. This is only temporary, of course, and it does nothing to stop catabolism. The bad cortisol hormone will continue to send this signal to eat up this hard-earned lean mass until you get real nutrients into your system.

It's important that breakfast include protein *and* carbohydrates *and* good fats *and* fiber.

Add a small glass of diluted unsweetened fruit juice to make a complete breakfast. The key here is unsweetened, since so many fruit juices are processed and loaded with high-fructose corn syrup and shamelessly marketed as nutritious.

Instead of drinking juice that's been fortified with sugar, why not eat the original fruit? Why not eat an orange instead of drinking a glass of orange juice? There's nothing wrong with orange juice, of course, but it's going to give you a higher glycemic response than the piece of fruit. Better to water it down or consume it with other foods that will lower the glycemic response.

But if you eat the orange, you get the added fiber and nutrients. The benefit is far superior to a glass of juice. Let your body be the manufacturing plant, squeezing out all the nutrients from an orange. Otherwise, the plant just grinds out the nutrients, sometimes adds sugar, and leaves you with a far inferior breakfast drink.

PIZZA FOR BREAKFAST? ■

When I started as a performance coach 15 years ago, I dealt mostly with college athletes. Like most college kids—and kids in general—they tended to skip breakfast, opting to sleep a few extra minutes before class in the morning rather than getting up in time to go to the dining hall or fixing a bowl of cereal in their apartments.

I tried everything to get them to eat breakfast. In a last-ditch effort, I said, "If I could just get you to eat a slice of cold pizza. . . ."

That got their attention. If nothing else, they finally understood the importance of breakfast once I was willing to let them eat pizza. A few of them did occasionally eat pizza, but they mostly made a concerted effort to eat something more nutritious.

I'd rather have you eat a piece of cold pizza, which usually is about 35 percent fat and 25 percent protein, than go without breakfast. Better to give the body something than remain in a semifasted state, with little energy.

College kids eat a lot of pizza. After all, most go to school without cooking skills, and the easiest option is to call Domino's or Pizza Hut. Adults, too, rely on pizza as a regular quick-food option.

If you're going to eat pizza on days other than your Sundays "off," do what you can to make it a healthier alternative. Start by ordering thin or "hand-tossed" crust, with tomato sauce and nutritious toppings. Pineapple, for instance, has good digestive enzymes. Spinach is loaded with nutrients. The tomato paste itself has antioxidant properties. Canadian bacon, ham, and chicken are good sources of protein. Black olives and olive oil are healthy fats. Even a light coating of cheese is a source of protein.

Avoid thick-crust, deep-dish, and stuffed-crust pizza. Blot off the extra grease with a napkin. Go easy on the cheese and avoid fatty toppings such as pepperoni, sausage, and ground beef. Drink water instead of beer or soft drinks.

Understand, I'm not recommending pizza as a solution for your nutrition program. But since it might be part of your lifestyle, take action to make sure it's as nutritious as possible. Above all else, the Core Nutrition Plan is about making the best choice in every situation, even if it involves pizza.

And even if you must eat it for breakfast.

COACHING KEY NO. 7: FOR LUNCH AND DINNER, THINK COMBO

The number one thing to remember when planning lunch and dinner, as with breakfast, is to have a combination of protein and carbs, preferably with plenty of fiber in both. Your diet is balanced, and the different foods will balance each other to produce maximum energy, build lean mass, and regulate your blood sugar level.

When you look at your plate, you should

see a lean protein source and some brightly colored carbs that are rich in fiber. You want to have some good fat, either from olive oil or fish.

As with breakfast, there's a tendency in our culture to skip lunch or eat something on the run that inevitably offers poor nutritional value. A deli sandwich on sourdough, pumpernickel, or rye is a great lunch. If you use mayonnaise, go with low-fat or fat-free, being careful to check the sugar and high-fructose corn syrup content. Try to use healthier condiments such as hummus, mustard, or horseradish.

A burrito also is a good lunch. Black beans are high in fiber and protein and low in fat. You can add chicken, tomatoes, and lettuce. Even guacamole is a good, unsaturated fat, comparable to olive oil. The tortilla is the worst part of the mix, since it's highly processed and creates too-large portions. A better option would be to put all the ingredients of the burrito on a bed of lettuce, creating a salad. (I highly recommend this burrito "salad bowl" at Chipotle, a growing national chain of restaurants that serves nutritious Mexican food. In fact, I often worked on this book while eating there.)

A can of tuna on whole wheat bread or with lettuce is a quality lunch. And keep in mind that anything that can be placed on bread can be made into a salad to improve its nutritional value. With any lunch, make sure you include vegetables for a complete, nutritious meal.

Lunch and dinner need not be major productions, especially since you're eating more often. If you take some fish, chicken, or lean red meat; add some vegetables, fruit, or both; and wash it down with two glasses of cold water, or even a glass of red wine, you have a good meal.

As we mentioned earlier, for convenience you can cook plenty of chicken and fish on Sundays. Buy some prepackaged salads. Put together some vegetables and fruits. The key is to have things ready so you won't be left hungry and scrambling for food, which inevitably will result in a poor nutritional choice.

COACHING KEY NO. 8: BETWEEN-MEAL SNACKS ARE A GOOD THING

From a young age, many of us were taught to avoid eating between meals. We'll get fat and, at the very least, spoil our dinners. At least that's what a generation of parents led us to believe.

Actually, spoiling dinner is not such a bad thing if it means you won't overeat, as most people do. By eating often, as we discussed earlier, you keep adding wood to the fire, and it burns hotter and faster. You need to keep your blood sugar levels consistent to minimize overeating. The only way to do this is to eat every 2½ to 3 hours.

As with your meals, you want your snacks to include a combination of high-fiber carbohydrates, proteins, and fats. You could have a cup of low-fat cottage cheese or low-fat yogurt (with no added sugar). You could have a piece of fruit with natural peanut butter, or a handful of nuts. Beef jerky is a good snack. A little tuna or chicken combined with a fruit or vegetable also works.

For some people, there might be little difference between their meals and snacks. Your breakfasts, lunches, and dinners might be smaller than what you've traditionally eaten, since you no longer are trying to eat enough to contain your appetite for the next 6 to 12 hours.

Then again, the size of your meals might remain consistent, with your snacks being somewhat modest. That's okay, too, as long as your snacks contain protein, high-fiber carbs, and good fats. For time and convenience, you might want to have a protein shake or a higher-protein meal-replacement bar.

The challenge with meal-replacement bars is to find something that tastes good and is good for you. Look at the label carefully. Your goal is to find something with 15 to 30 grams of protein, 8 to 20 grams of carbs, and a few grams of fat. These include the EAS Advant-Edge bar, the Met-Rx Protein-Plus bars, Detour bars, and the Balance Bar line.

You have snacks and shakes built into your schedule three times a day. You might find the late-afternoon feeding the most important, since people tend to feel most sluggish at that time.

For the night feeding, you'll want something that's going to stick with you, since it will be a long time before you eat again. Some chicken or fish left over from dinner would be a good snack. Or a protein shake. Or a green apple with peanut butter. Look for something with plenty of fiber.

So don't feel guilty about those between-meal snacks. In fact, look at them not as guilty pleasures but as essential components to a healthy lifestyle.

COACHING KEY NO. 9: MAKE SUPPLEMENTATION A DAILY RITUAL

Walk into any health food store or General Nutrition Center (GNC), and you'll find a dizzying array of powders, capsules, and drinks that promise to transform your body. For simplicity, we're not going to bother with most of them in this book.

You already know that I recommend a preworkout shooter or postworkout recovery mix, and shakes as snacks up to two additional times per day. It's also a good idea to take a multivitamin in the morning or evening, along with an antioxidant complex, which is chock-full of vitamins and minerals.

Brightly colored foods usually are powerful

APPROVED SUPPLEMENTS ■

As the director of performance for the NFL Players Association, I want to make sure this area is safe not only for players but also for the public. We're developing a certification program, an elaborate process with very stringent requirements, that will place an accreditation label on supplements to let consumers know that the product contains what's on the label and that it's free of banned substances. Just because something is legal doesn't mean that it's approved by the major sports organizations or that it meets any scientific or manufacturing criteria.

Rather than waiting for the Food and Drug Administration to determine what products might be contaminated or spiked purposely with bad substances, we're taking a proactive approach to supplements. Look for our labels early in 2004.

antioxidants. If you're eating well, following this program, you can get by without antioxidant supplementation. But even elite athletes who come to Athletes' Performance and have their blood analyzed almost always are found to be deficient in some antioxidants.

Here's why. Whenever our bodies endure stress—whether it's from physical activity, sun damage, pollution, or day-to-day family and job stresses—we suffer cellular damage. It's unavoidable. Those damaged cells are known as free radicals. We want to minimize their impact and get them out of our system immediately.

Think of free radicals as unruly nightclub patrons. Antioxidants are the bouncers that escort them out. They maintain order among your cells and slow the aging process. They're critical to your immediate and long-term health. You can find a bottle of antioxidants at a health food store, supermarket, or Wal-Mart for about

$5 and up. We recommend a product called Vitrin to our athletes. Though more expensive than run-of-the-mill antioxidants, two Vitrin caplets contain 29 essential vitamins and minerals, plus the antioxidant equivalent of five servings of fruits and vegetables.

There's been a lot of concern in recent years about supplements, much of it well-deserved. There's stuff you can buy legally in a health food store that I strongly urge our athletes never to take, either because of anecdotal evidence that suggests it's harmful or because no long-term studies have been conducted on the effects. I recommend that you stick to the supplemental foods recommended in this book.

The preworkout shooters, along with the workout recovery mixes I recommend as snacks or postworkout meals, are simply convenient liquid food: combinations of proteins and carbs with essential vitamins and minerals. Some

DON'T DRINK CALORIES ■

If you want to reduce calories quickly, cut them out of your drinks. If you replace soft drinks, juices, sports drinks, and beer with water or a "fitness water" like Gatorade Propel or Amino Vital, you'll cut down on calories and sugar. Without those calories for energy, your body will burn the higher-fiber carbs you're eating in the Core Nutrition Plan for energy. You'll lose fat and probably weight, too. For convenience, buy a case of bottled water and keep the bottles nearby in the refrigerator. That way you're more likely to grab water instead of sugary drinks.

contain fiber and good fats. They're conveniently packaged so they give you the best bang for your buck before or after exercise. If you're going to put so much effort into working out, it's vital that you optimize the recovery process.

You don't need a blender to fix a shake. Take a packet of shake mix, put it in a large plastic cup with cold water, cover, and shake thoroughly. (You can even buy a convenient plastic shake bottle for less than $10 at a health food store or through www.coreperformance.com.) If that's not easy enough, you now can buy a ready-to-drink mix in a can.

Remember that you've already done the hard part by working out. It takes only a moment to down that shake and start realizing the benefit.

COACHING KEY NO. 10: STAY HYDRATED

If I said that you could do up to 25 percent more work or run 25 percent farther, you'd sprint through a wall to make that happen, right? Actually, it's much easier. Just drink enough water before, during, and after exercise. Drink a gallon of water a day. Drink 2 cups of water first thing in the morning. Take a big gallon jug to work and drink all day. Keep a bottle in the car.

Recent research suggests that *any* beverage, even one with caffeine, promotes hydration, but there's still nothing better than water.

Water has a direct impact on the aging process. Because of dehydration, inactivity, and trauma from daily life, the connective tissues around our muscles and joints dry up over time, sort of like those chew toys for dogs that start out soft and pliable and end up stiff and brittle. Just drinking sufficient water goes a long way toward preventing this process while improving your muscle tissue and flexibility.

Why drink caffeinated beverages when there's a perfect, healthier alternative available? Some people rationalize drinking diet soft drinks because the beverages have no

URINE COLOR/HYDRATION CHART

Use this chart to help determine hydration status.

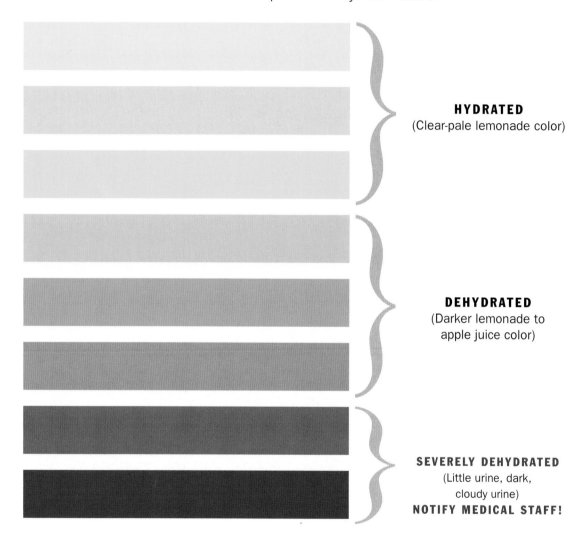

HYDRATED
(Clear-pale lemonade color)

DEHYDRATED
(Darker lemonade to
apple juice color)

SEVERELY DEHYDRATED
(Little urine, dark,
cloudy urine)
NOTIFY MEDICAL STAFF!

calories. That's true, but they still can damage your teeth and offer no nutritional value. We'd never put the automotive equivalent of diet soft drinks in our cars, but we do it to our bodies all the time.

As far as artificial sweeteners in soft drinks and other beverages go, recent research suggests that *modest* consumption of artificial sweeteners is a better alternative to high-fructose corn syrup and other sugars. Although

SUMMARY: CREATING A CHAMPIONSHIP MEAL STRATEGY ■

1. Eat smaller portions more often, spread evenly across the day.

2. Your carbohydrate intake should be relative to your activity level. Eat "glycemically correct" carbs, high in color and fiber. The less processed the better.

3. Select a lean protein source with each meal, along with some "fabulous" fats.

4. Choose carbs that are rich in fiber.

5. Drink a preworkout shooter or a postworkout recovery shake.

6. Add a multivitamin and antioxidant complex to your daily routine.

7. Stay hydrated.

8. Eat breakfast every day.

9. Eat a rainbow often, and the less legs, the better!

10. Mix foods for variety, nutrient density, and glycemic response.

I'm not a fan of diet soft drinks—it is better to drink water—I'd much rather see you drink a diet than a regular soft drink that's loaded with sugar. (A typical can has about 150 calories, all from sugar.)

If you drink coffee, don't overdo the cream and sugar. Again, this goes back to making healthier choices. Consider a healthier alternative such as green, white, or other teas, which have antioxidant properties.

There's no downside to water. If you drink too much, what's the worst that will happen? You'll sweat or excrete it out.

Proper hydration regulates appetite. A lot of times people think they're hungry when they're really just thirsty. If you're trying to lose weight, have a glass of water before eating, and you'll have that satiety that keeps you from overeating.

People tend to think it's impossible to drink a gallon of water a day. These often are the same people who have 3 cups of coffee in the morning, a couple of diet soft drinks with lunch, and alcoholic beverages during and after dinner. They all provide hydration, but are not nearly as healthy as water.

If you substitute water, you'll have no problem drinking a gallon a day. Drink two glasses when you wake up, two glasses with every meal, and plenty of water before, during, and after working out. If you're training hard, especially in warmer climates, you may find you actually exceed a gallon a day.

You probably won't miss the caffeine. The Core Nutrition Plan helps you regulate your blood sugar and maintain your energy level, so you won't feel the need to use caffeine as an artificial energy source.

Don't assume that sports drinks are an equal substitute for water, especially for people in everyday life. In fact, most are loaded with a ton of high-glycemic carbohydrates that elevate blood sugar and ultimately contribute to body fat.

Sports drinks are most valuable for endurance athletes competing in prolonged, intense activity. These athletes need to replace sugars immediately. But most of us never reach that level of exertion.

How do you know if you're properly hydrated? Take a look at your urine. Generally speaking, the clearer the urine, the better hydrated you are. We've even included a handy reference chart on page 223.

For some reason, these charts are very popular at Athletes' Performance. Since men like to have something to read in the bathroom, we post them above the urinals, not unlike how restaurants tack up advertisements or newspapers. (They're posted in the women's rooms, too.)

Throughout this program, I want you to get better in tune with your body. Develop a better sense of how it operates and what affects it. Measuring your hydration level is one easy way.

You might want to make color copies of this page and keep them in the bathrooms in your home. You'll find it's impossible *not* to look at the charts. I've had athletes tell me they've used the chart to help potty-train their kids, who inevitably find it amusing to compare the color of their urine to a chart.

Whatever works, right? Seriously, it's never too early to get into the habit of drinking an adequate amount of water. And if you've been living on caffeine, soft drinks, and alcohol, it's never too late to change.

CHAPTER 14

CORE PERFORMANCE FOODS

Embarking on a new diet plan is always a challenge. After all, we're creatures of habit. We go into a grocery store and roll down the aisles on autopilot, grabbing the same foods we've eaten for years. But if we take just a moment and consider some healthier alternatives, many of which taste better, we can change our lives. We'll look and feel better, have more energy, and live longer.

When you go grocery shopping, work the perimeter. Virtually everything you need is along the outer aisles, such as produce, fish, meat, and dairy products. Instead of going down every aisle, glance at the overhead signs to locate healthy items like canned tuna fish, oatmeal, and olive oil. Leave the cart at one end and walk down the aisle. That way you avoid being tempted by cake mixes, cookies, chips, and soft drinks. And, as a bonus, you'll save time.

The foods in the table on page 228—categorized as "good," "neutral," or "bad"—should include many of your favorites. I understand that you're sometimes going to eat certain foods regardless of nutritional value; all of us have a few of these that are part of our lifestyle or family traditions. You might also enjoy some healthy foods not on the list, and of course that's great. Consider this list a mere starting point.

You may be surprised by some of the foods classified as "neutral" or "bad." Many times, foods are marketed as nutritious and healthy when in reality they aren't. Meanwhile, some of the best foods go unnoticed simply because they're not manufactured by companies with huge advertising budgets.

Unfortunately, most of us learn about foods from the worst possible sources—the

(continued on page 230)

THE BEST AND WORST FOODS
(AND EVERYTHING IN BETWEEN)

FATS

Good	**Oils and sprays:** Canola oil, canola spray, Enova oil, fish oil, flaxseed oil, I Can't Believe It's Not Butter spray, olive oil (extra virgin), olive oil spray (extra virgin), Benecol Spread **Vegetables:** Avocadoes **Seeds:** Pumpkin, sunflower **Nuts:** Almonds, cashews, macadamias, pecans, soy nuts, walnuts
Neutral	**Nuts:** Natural peanut butter, peanuts
Bad	**Dairy products:** Butter, cream, ice cream (regular, full-fat), margarine, milk (whole) **Oils:** Lard (Crisco, etc.)

PROTEINS

Good	**Fish:** Anchovies, calamari, cod, flounder, grouper, halibut, mackerel, mahi mahi, salmon (wild over farm-raised), sardines, swordfish, tuna (canned in water), tuna steak or sushi **Shellfish:** Clams/mussels, crab, lobster, oysters, shrimp/prawns **Poultry:** Chicken breast (skinless), ground turkey (extra-lean), turkey breast **Meat:** Buffalo, filet mignon, flank steak, ground beef (93% lean), ham (96% fat-free), London broil, pork loin (lean), top and bottom round, venison **Legumes:** Black beans, soybeans (edamame) **Dairy products:** Cheeses (less than 2% fat), Egg Beaters, egg whites, milk (fat-free—skim), yogurt (low-fat, low-sugar)
Neutral	**Poultry:** Chicken (dark meat, skinless), ground turkey (85–90% lean) **Meat:** Ground beef (85–90% lean), roast beef **Legumes (eaten alone):** Chickpeas, kidney beans, lentils, pinto beans **Dairy products:** Cottage cheese (1% and 2% fat), frozen yogurt (low-fat, low-sugar), ice cream (low-fat/fat-free, low-sugar), milk (1% and 2% fat), whole eggs, yogurt (whole milk)
Bad	**Meat:** Beef (heavily marbled), ground beef (regular fat), NY strip, T-bone, chicken (with skin or fried) **Dairy products:** Cheeses (double- or triple-cream, such as Brie and Camembert), milk (whole)

CARBOHYDRATES

Good	***Breads:*** Pumpernickel, rye, sourdough
	Cereals: Cheerios, Kashi, oatmeal (slow-cooking—not instant)
	Starches: Brown rice, couscous, quinoa
	Root vegetables: Beets, sweet potatoes, yams
	Green vegetables: Asparagus, broccoli, brussel sprouts, cucumber, field greens, green beans, romaine lettuce, snap peas, spinach
	Other vegetables: Bell peppers, carrots, celery, eggplant, mushrooms, soybeans squash, tomatoes
	Fruit: Apples (green), blackberries, blueberries, cantaloupe, cherries, grapefruit, grapes (red), honeydew, kiwifruit, mangoes, oranges (whole), papaya, peaches, plums, pomegranates, raspberries, strawberries, watermelon
Neutral	***Breads and baked goods:*** Bread (whole wheat), muffins (oat or whole wheat), tortillas (whole wheat)
	Cereals: Corn-based cereals (all), rice-based cereals (all)
	Starches: Egg noodles, pancakes (nonenriched/ whole wheat, buckwheat, or sourdough—no-/low-sugar syrup), pasta (whole wheat or vegetable)
	Root vegetables: Potatoes (baked)
	Other vegetables: Iceberg lettuce, yellow squash, zucchini
	Fruit: Dates
	Snacks: English muffins (sourdough), rice cakes, wheat crackers
Bad	***Baked goods:*** Cakes, cookies, doughnuts, English muffins (most types), white bread
	Cereals: Sugary cereals
	Dairy products: Frozen yogurt (with sugar), ice cream
	Snacks/treats: Dried fruit, french fries, granola bars, potato chips, trail mix
	Salads: Coleslaw, creamy seafood salad, potato salad

(continued)

THE BEST AND WORST FOODS (CONT.)
(AND EVERYTHING IN BETWEEN)

BEVERAGES

Good	Red wine (2–6 glasses per week), tea (decaffeinated—green, black, or white), water (at least 64 oz. per day)
Neutral	Coffee (decaf or regular), diet soft drinks, fruit juices (unsweetened), orange juice (diluted), teas (caffeinated), white wine
Bad	Beer, fruit juice (sweetened), hard liquor, Kool-Aid, mixed drinks (especially fruity bar drinks), smoothies, soft drinks, wine coolers

CONDIMENTS

Good	Balsamic vinegar, Benecol spread, cayenne pepper, fruit spreads, garlic, herbs/spices, horseradish, hummus, mayonnaise (fat-free), Mrs. Dash seasoning, mustard, pesto, salad dressing (fat-free), salsa, seasonings, Take Control spread
Neutral	BBQ sauce, ketchup, salad dressing (low-fat), syrup (light)
Bad	Mayonnaise, Miracle Whip, salad dressing (regular), sugar

media and advertising. Much of this information is inaccurate, and what isn't inaccurate is almost always incomplete. You have to fill in the blanks. Examine labels for content, especially the amounts of proteins, fats, and carbs. If you're good with numbers, try to calculate the percentages of each in the food. Look at the line that tells you how many grams of sugar are in the product, then look at the list of ingredients to see what kind of sugar it is. I've already explained that high-fructose corn syrup (or HFCS) is to be avoided. Same with fat—if you see the word *hydrogenated,* that means it's a trans fat and another ingredient you want to avoid whenever possible.

All this reading and calculating might take a few extra minutes at first, but pretty soon you'll be able to cruise through the aisles— maybe even faster than before.

Don't let some slick marketing campaign dictate what you're going to eat and drink. After all, no one believes (I hope) that smoking cigarettes and drinking a lot of beer are going to improve your appearance, health, and quality of life, but there was a time when advertising shamelessly told you they would.

Now let's go aisle by aisle through the supermarket and help you fill your grocery cart with high-quality *Core Performance* foods.

PRODUCE

It's hard to go wrong in this section of the grocery store. Since we're looking to "eat a rainbow often," we should fill up a good chunk of our cart right here. I call produce such as tomatoes, blueberries, spinach, asparagus, broccoli, and pomegranates "power foods" because they're rich in color, fiber, and antioxidant properties.

When choosing fruits and vegetables, fresh or fresh-frozen is the best way to go. Frozen fruits and veggies are preferable to canned goods since nutrients are lost in the canning process. Frozen can be preferable to fresh if there's any chance the fresh food will go bad before you get to finish it.

Avoid dried fruits and trail mixes, which are calorie dense and too heavy in sugar.

Fruit and vegetable platters are healthy alternatives to chips and dips to serve at parties.

DELI

You always want to go for the leanest cuts of meat possible. When selecting turkey, ham, and chicken, go for a brand that's at least 97 percent fat-free.

Prepackaged salads are convenient and save time. Garden salads are fine, provided the dressing is on the side. Go easy on the croutons. As always, the more color to your salad, the better. Salads with leafy spinach and romaine lettuce tend to be more colorful than those made predominantly with iceberg lettuce. Stay away from potato salad and other creamy side dishes.

Rotisserie chicken is one of my favorites. It's flavorful, precooked, and it provides several meals out of a single chicken at an affordable price. The key is to drain the fat, remove the fatty skin, and pat the bird down with a paper towel.

When you eat cheese, do so in moderation—ideally, treat it as a garnish. Go for low-fat, semisoft cheeses. Generally speaking, softer cheeses are better.

BREAD AND BAKED GOODS

There's little nutritional value to be found in this aisle, since you want to avoid processed foods. When you must eat bread, opt for a less-processed type, such as pumpernickel, rye, sourdough, or whole wheat. You want to see words in the label that indicate that whole grain flour is the main ingredient. Don't be fooled by loaves of brown bread labeled as "wheat." If it's not made with whole wheat flour, it's just white bread dyed to look like something more nutritious.

With wheat bread, look for "stone-ground" or "crushed wheat" on the label. Whole wheat breads marketed as "light" generally tend to come in thinner slices, which is another way to keep from overdoing it on breads. Avoid white, buttermilk, or split-top "wheat" breads; they have too much enriched flour (the stuff that's been heavily processed). Be on the lookout for high-fructose corn syrup; it even appears in bread.

Bagels and English muffins should be eaten only in the morning and with the proper toppings (natural peanut butter, light cream cheese, and so forth).

As for tortillas, one has as much as 40 grams of carbs and could be very high in fat. If you must have one, go for a whole wheat version.

Skip the cake mixes, muffins, brownies, and doughnuts—pretty much the entire baked goods aisle.

CONDIMENTS AND JELLIES

Spend some time reading the labels in this aisle. Whether it's salad dressing, barbecue sauce, ketchup, or mayonnaise, it's important to examine the grams of fat and sugar and the number of calories per serving. High-fructose corn syrup rears its ugly head often in this area.

I'm not a big fan of mayonnaise, but if you must have it, go with a brand that's low in fat and carbs. Mustard, hummus, salsa, and horseradish are better alternatives.

Hummus (pronounced HUM-iss) is an exotic blend of lemon, chickpeas, garlic, sesame puree, and olive oil that contains no saturated fat, cholesterol, or sugar. It also contains protein and fiber. Unlike a lot of so-called health foods, hummus tastes great. Use it on sandwiches instead of mayonnaise. It also works well on fish and chicken.

Salad dressings can be deceiving. One manufacturer's "low-fat" version might be comparable to the standard brand of another company. Whatever kind you choose, go easy on the dressing once you start using it at home. Consider mixing olive oil and balsamic vinegar for a tasty alternative. Extra-virgin olive oil is preferable; it's produced from the first pressing of olives and has less than 1 percent acidity.

It also pays to eyeball the jelly and jam labels. The lower the sugar content, the better. Straight fruit spreads (as opposed to preserves) are preferable.

Peanut butter sometimes gets a bad rap. Natural peanut butter is far better than your run-of-the-mill creamy brands. Natural peanut butter has oil floating at the top. Pour off about half of it and mix up the rest. If you must go with a standard peanut butter, be careful with the reduced-fat products. Manufacturers tend to pour in the high-fructose corn syrup.

Speaking of butter, skip it. Instead, try a low-fat, low-calorie substitute like I Can't Believe It's Not Butter. The spray is preferable to the tub, since there's a tendency to go overboard with spreads. You get better coverage and use less with the spray. Olive oil, Enova oil, or Pam cooking spray, made from canola oil, is ideal for cooking.

Spices such as oregano and parsley are a great way to get flavor without adding lots of calories. Spice blends made specifically for seafood, salads, or meat make it convenient to add flavor. Remove sugar from the house and replace it with Splenda, a no-calorie sweetener that's made from sugar but doesn't have the bitter aftertaste of artificial sweeteners.

CEREALS AND BREAKFAST FOODS

Besides being ridiculously expensive, many cereals provide only modest nutritional value. Too often they're loaded with sugar and calories.

The 5-minute version of old-fashioned Quaker Oats has been around forever but is still arguably the best breakfast cereal option.

The 1-minute version and the prepackaged products are more processed.

The original Cheerios also is a good choice since it, too, is made from oats. Avoid the sugary versions of Cheerios.

I'm a big fan of the cereals and other foods made by Kashi. This company has been around since 1984, though most people still have not heard of it. Kashi makes a pilaf product with seven whole grains. It can be used as a hot breakfast meal or a nutritious side dish for lunch or dinner. The company also makes waffles that are high in fiber and an excellent breakfast choice.

At the risk of sounding like a Kashi spokesman, I like the company's philosophy outlined on its Web site. Kashi believes "that everyone has the power to make healthful changes . . . to make the right changes to reach your health, wellness, and weight-management goals with all-natural foods that are minimally processed and free of highly refined sugars, unnecessary additives, and preservatives." That's a great strategy. No matter what food you select, it's hard to go wrong if you choose based on minimal processing and an absence of sugars and preservatives.

Pancakes are permissible so long as you don't make a complete meal out of them. There's nothing wrong with having *one* pancake with, say, an egg-white omelet. Use I Can't Believe It's Not Butter spray instead of butter on your pancake. Use syrup sparingly and look for brands with low or no sugar. Not surprisingly, syrup often is loaded with high-fructose corn syrup.

Egg whites or similar substitutes are preferable to eggs. For those times when you do bake, consider replacing eggs partially or fully with egg whites. (Two egg whites are equivalent to one egg.) Again, make the best choice possible, even if you're eating cake.

FISH AND MEAT

Remember the rule: The less legs, the better. It's tough to go wrong with fish, though it should be baked, grilled, or broiled—never fried or breaded.

Salmon is one of my top power foods. Besides being a better source of protein than most meats, it's loaded with omega-3 fatty acids, which have heart disease–reducing properties. It's probably no coincidence that Japan consumes the highest amount of salmon per person and has among the lowest levels of heart disease in the world. Not only that, many people find salmon more flavorful than other fish.

Shrimp, crab, lobster, clams, and calamari are nutritious foods as long as they're not fried or mixed into creamy seafood salads. Canned tuna fish is an excellent source of protein; just make sure it's canned in water, not vegetable oil. Tuna fish is now available in handy tear-open foil packs as well.

After fish, chicken and poultry have the fewest legs. Some people, like former big-league baseball player Wade Boggs, can eat chicken every day. Cornish game hens are a good alternative, though like chicken they should be stripped of skin. As with fish, poultry never should be fried or breaded.

Contrary to popular belief, lean red meat is great for you. Lean cuts are high in protein, low in fat, and great sources of iron, phosphorus, and creatine. Red meat should be consumed in moderation, but there's no reason to eliminate it from your diet. When selecting a cut, go lean. The less "marbling," or fat, the better.

A good strategy is to select cuts made from the animal's muscles of locomotion. Top and bottom round are lean cuts, since they come from rear legs of the animal. They're named for the round bone of the femur. Flank cuts also are very lean, and a cube steak is very lean. Avoid fattier, more marbled cuts such as strips, fillets, and T-bones. Lean pork is a great, nutritious alternative.

PASTA AND SIDE DISHES

Many diets prohibit pasta altogether. The key to pasta is to look at it as a side dish, not as an entire meal. A small, fist-size serving of pasta—preferably whole wheat or vegetable pasta—is acceptable. Go with low-sugar, meatless pasta sauce, or make your own, adding extra-lean ground beef or turkey.

When choosing rice, go with brown or wild, since it's less processed and has more fiber than white rice. A better alternative to rice is couscous. Pronounced "koos-koos," it's a staple of North African cooking and is made from durum wheat, the ideal pasta wheat because of its high protein content.

Soybeans are another power food. They're rich in nutrients and high in protein.

SWEETS AND MEAL-REPLACEMENT BARS

It may seem impossible for you to go a day without having sweets. Like everything else, though, you can make better choices if you try. You might get your fix with some sweet fruits. If not, try a low-sugar frozen-fruit bar. If you're a chocoholic, go with a fat-free Fudgsicle, which is low in sugar and has just 60 calories.

When choosing ice cream, look for brands that are low in fat and sugar. (A fat-free brand might be heavy in high-fructose corn syrup.) Buy small containers of ice cream, since studies suggest that the larger the container, the larger the serving a person will take. This seems obvious, but think about it. If you have a brand new half-gallon container, you'll probably think nothing of scooping out 8 to 10 ounces of ice cream. But if you have a smaller container, you'll probably take less, not wanting to look or feel like a pig.

Yogurt can be tricky. A fat-free yogurt might have a lot of sugar calories. It's also better to take a plain yogurt and mix your own fruit in than to eat yogurt with (processed) fruit on the bottom. It's generally a good bet to go with a low-sugar, low-fat yogurt. Add in some fiber with oats, nuts, seeds, or a teaspoon of flaxseed or fish oil.

The same rules apply to frozen yogurt. Yogurt stores generally provide a breakdown of the fat and sugar content of their products.

Meal-replacement bars can be a good late-afternoon "meal." Unfortunately, many bars have the same nutritional value as candy bars. Ideally, a meal-replacement bar should have a carbs-to-protein ratio of no more than 2:1—generally, the more protein, the better. So if a bar has 30 grams of carbs, it should have at least 15 grams of protein. Many new products have a higher ratio of protein, such as 1:2, meaning 15 grams of carbs and 30 grams of protein.

Avoid granola bars, which tend to be highly processed, calorically dense, and high in sugar.

Individual preferences vary widely when it comes to meal-replacement bars. Bars you find delicious might taste like chalk or cardboard to someone else. If you've had bad experiences with meal-replacement bars in the past, give them another chance. You'll be amazed at how much better they taste. Some even taste like candy bars.

BEVERAGES

Water, of course, is the ideal beverage. Pick up a case of 12- or 16-ounce bottles to take to work, the gym, or your car when you're out running errands. If you live in an area with poor-quality water, buy gallon jugs of distilled water.

Unless you're a serious endurance athlete, someone who's involved in running, biking, or other strenuous activities for long periods of time, you probably don't need anything more than water or "fitness water." You definitely don't need regular sports drinks for routine refreshment around the house or at work. (Remember: Don't drink calories!) If you're looking for added taste, try a fitness water like Gatorade Propel or Amino Vital.

When choosing sports drinks, make sure they don't contain high-fructose corn syrup, a standard ingredient in most soft drinks. Avoid the self-serve soda fountains at restaurants unless you're going for the water, which incidentally is highly filtered and purified.

If you must have soft drinks, go with a diet beverage. I'm not advocating diet soft drinks by any means—giving up soft drinks might be the easiest way for you to get more water—but if you must have them, find a diet brand you like. They will keep you hydrated, but water still is the best choice.

Be careful when choosing fruit juice, which often contains too much sugar and high-fructose corn syrup. Always look on the label at the percentage of fruit juice to sugar. Most juice can be diluted further with water, which lowers its glycemic load. You'll also get more out of it, which is a good thing since juice, like cereal, is one of those items that's ridiculously overpriced.

For many people, life is impossible without their daily coffee. The *Core Performance* program, including proper sleep, should wean you away from caffeine addiction. When you do drink coffee, don't overdo the cream and sugar.

Green tea is a great substitute for coffee. I call it a "power drink," since it's a natural source of antioxidants. If you must have sugar with your coffee or tea, go with Splenda.

Fat-free milk or 1% is better than whole or 2%, which is a rule that applies to all dairy products.

By now, your shopping cart should be bulging with foods that taste great and have tremendous nutritional value. The biggest misperception about eating right is that your meals have to be bland and boring, with very little flavor. Nothing could be further from the truth. By using just the items suggested throughout this chapter, you could produce dozens of rich, tasty meals.

How do I know? Well, not only do I follow this diet myself, but the athletes that train at Athletes' Performance do as well. I know that if I didn't provide them with tasty food options, they wouldn't stick to the program. Many of them have the financial means to eat every breakfast, lunch, and dinner at the best restaurants in town.

Instead, they eat at our café, where Debbie Martell, our performance chef, makes meals that adhere to the Core Nutrition Plan. Her meals taste so good that athletes often look at her dishes suspiciously, thinking they look and taste far too good to be nutritious.

Debbie has 15 years' experience as a chef, along with a degree in nutrition and dietetics. But you don't need any of those credentials to put together some of her favorite recipes. Be sure to check them out at www.coreperformance.com.

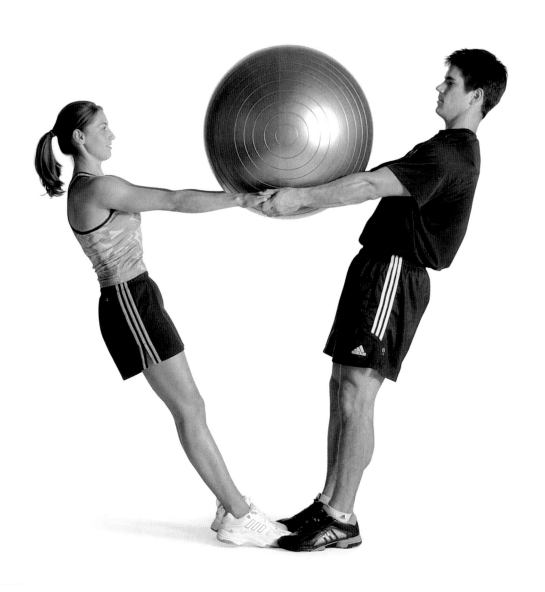

PART

4

THE CORE
LIFE PLAN

CHAPTER 15

THE CORE CHALLENGE (REVISITED)

My friend and colleague Darryl Eto is fond of saying that I have the ability to *will* people to get better. That's very flattering, but I prefer to think of my role as one of showing people how they can become better on their own.

I'm honored that you've chosen me to be your performance coach, and I believe that the programs and philosophies in these pages will inspire and motivate you to pursue excellence, not just in the physical realm but also in other areas of your life.

Ultimately, it's going to be your decision to embark on this journey. It will be a challenge, no question about it. Finding the time and the discipline to adhere to anything can be difficult, and I admire you for making the commitment.

This is where you draw the line in the sand. Are you going to remain at the status quo, or are you going to make a commitment and decision to see what you're capable of achieving? Make the decision now that you're going to obtain those goals for yourself and your family.

After all, you'll have to face the results of your decision now or later, and the alternative to not making the commitment to live your dreams every day is the painful realization that you haven't lived your life to the fullest. Remember, I'm not asking much more here than what others have recommended. The Surgeon General and American College of Sports Medicine suggest a minimum of 30 minutes of exercise a day—just 3 percent of your waking time. All I'm doing is showing you how to maximize the value of that time.

As you follow the *Core Performance* plan, as you weave the core philosophies throughout your life, you'll not only experience tremendous physical benefits—your entire outlook on life will improve, too. You'll come to understand that you can overcome any obstacle or challenge and obtain any goal in every part of your life.

If this were only a physical program, it would be easy to stop at a certain point. You might lose a few pounds, gain lean muscle mass and flexibility, and feel great about yourself for a while.

Don't get me wrong, those are awesome accomplishments. But too many people treat a new training regimen as a short-term goal. They want to lose some weight or have more energy. They want to look better at the beach.

All of those things are admirable, and they will happen if you follow this program. But don't miss the opportunity to use this as a springboard to transform your life and the lives of those around you.

We've presented *Core Performance* as a 12-week plan, but I hope you'll realize the benefits and continue forward. As I mentioned in the preface to the Core Workout worksheets, you can turn up the intensity after 12 weeks. You also can look for advanced exercises on our Web site: www.coreperformance.com.

It would be a shame to quit at the end of 12 weeks, after making so much progress, or to return to one-dimensional exercise programs. Each of us has been given a set of gifts, and it's our responsibility to optimize those gifts throughout life. That's why I want you to spend 5 to 6 hours a week taking care of your physical well-being, time that you'll make the most of to make sure you get the best return on your investment.

By making this investment in yourself physically, you improve not only your health but also your mental and spiritual outlook. You become a better spouse, better parent, better sibling. That means the lives of your loved ones improve as well.

DREAMS AND GOALS

My most rewarding accomplishment is that I've been able to help people improve their lives. Some of those people are prominent athletes that you've heard from in this book, but many others are outside the limelight. I would never call them "normal" people because everyone has unique gifts and limitless potential. But when they started this program, they were everyday people with unrealized goals that they gradually had given up on as they became more caught up in the daily routine of work, paying bills, and just trying to keep up in a world that seems to move faster all the time. Now they've reached extraordinary levels of success.

Take a moment right now to write down five goals. Let the first goal be huge, something to accomplish in the next 5 years. The second should be something to accomplish in the next 2 years, and the third something for the next year. The fourth goal should be for the next 6 months, and the fifth for the next 3 months.

Dream big, but be specific and avoid physical and sport-specific goals since we listed those at the beginning of the book. (You did list those goals, right? If not, flip back to page 23 right now and list those goals before going any further.)

Now, back to those dreams. Think big picture. What is your perfect world? Do you want to start your own business? Change careers? Buy your own home? Move to a certain area of the country? Take a fabulous 3-week vacation each summer?

Kids, do you want to get into a certain college? Pursue a career in professional sports or entertainment? Study to become a doctor or a college professor? Maybe you want to start a business right now as a teenager.

Whatever your goals, no matter how outrageous they might seem, write them down immediately. Studies show that people who write down goals are more likely to achieve them, no matter how unlikely they might seem.

I'll give you an example from my own life. For many years, I had a dream of owning and operating a performance-training center that would cater to elite athletes. We would offer cutting-edge training methods based on scientific research to help athletes realize their dreams.

Not only that, but I wanted the facility to be independent, not influenced by investors or outside interests. I didn't want to have to answer to anyone other than my athlete clients or lose focus on their best interests.

Problem: I'm not independently wealthy. In 1999, when I moved to Phoenix, I was only a few years removed from the days when I earned a salary of $22,400 a year as an assistant director of player development at the Georgia Institute of Technology.

I wasn't sure where I would obtain the financing and how I could make this dream possible. I won't bore you with the details of how my colleagues and I were able to overcome numerous obstacles to build the multimillion-dollar business known as Athletes' Performance. But I will tell you this: The key was that I defined that goal, along with a few other personal goals, and focused on it on a daily basis. At the end of each day, I'd ask myself, "Did I make progress today toward my goals?" Some days I made more progress than other days, but each day I at least inched a little closer.

Once that feat was accomplished, I set the bar higher with loftier goals. We now have a second Athletes' Performance training facility in Carson, California, part of the Anschutz Entertainment Group's Home Depot Center, and have exciting new projects on the horizon. It all started by following not just the Core Workout but also the core principles outlined in this book. I adamantly believe that anyone set on the face of this earth can achieve whatever he or she wants, if that person has the right vision and the right goal and focuses on it professionally and personally. Once you have a plan of attack, you can accomplish anything.

Take a moment right now to write down your five goals. You can do it right here. Or make a copy of this page or write it somewhere else. Put the list someplace where it won't get lost, and where you'll see it frequently.

I've found it motivating to create a collage of photos that illustrate these goals. You could use family photos, pictures from magazines, personal sketches—anything that represents your dreams. Keep the collage near your list of goals; paste it to the back if you like.

Goal One (5 years):
——————————————————
——————————————————
——————————————————

Goal Two (2 years):
——————————————————
——————————————————
——————————————————

Goal Three (1 year):
——————————————————
——————————————————
——————————————————

Goal Four (6 months):
——————————————————
——————————————————
——————————————————

Goal Five (3 months):
——————————————————
——————————————————
——————————————————

While you're making plans, I want you to schedule a week, or at least a long weekend, to enjoy after the initial 12 weeks of this program are over. Go on vacation or at least do something pleasurable near home. Schedule this "reload" week now so that you can look forward to it daily and use it as inspiration to work harder.

Now that you have two sets of goals, along with a reload week on the calendar, I want you to make a third list, which I call action or "process" goals. There's great power in committing to goals that are not just end results but part of the process. For instance, setting a goal of losing 10 pounds is great, but if you set an action goal of avoiding high-fructose corn syrup or eating six small meals a day, you've created a powerful strategy to make it happen.

As you've read this book, you've probably thought certain elements are going to be more difficult to implement than others. Some elements might be more important for you depending on your health, fitness level, or schedule.

Take a minute and list five goals that will help you stay on track. Write the goals in the first person and make them positive. For instance, if you have tight hips, you could write, "I will do the Movement Prep routine four times a week." If you need to drink more water, then write, "I will drink one gallon of water a day."

These process goals could be something as simple as using olive oil and hummus as substitutes for mayonnaise and salad dressing. Or eating good-tasting meal-replacement bars with a high protein-to-carbs ratio instead of candy, chips, and cookies. Or drinking fewer calories. Maybe you thought you needed to avoid red meat. Instead, set a goal of eating lean red meat once or twice a week. Pledge to eat six times a day. Or do some hot and cold contrasts each time you shower.

Maybe time is your most pressing concern. You could promise to perform Movement Prep at least four times a week. Or do the Physioball Routine *Y*s, *T*s, *W*s, and *L*s after waking up each morning. Or, if nothing else, follow the abbreviated version of the Core Workout for time-crunched and frequent travelers on page 198. Don't stress out if you have to do abbreviated workouts or even miss a day. Just stay committed and focus on these goals every day.

Have some fun with this, but make sure your process-oriented goals will help you fulfill those broader sets of dreams you listed earlier.

Goal One:

_____

_____

_____

Goal Two:

_____

_____

_____

Goal Three:

_____

_____

_____

Goal Four:

_____

_____

_____

Goal Five:

_____

_____

_____

I've had great success supporting people in the pursuit of their dreams. Indeed, what I love most is being able to build people, to see them evolve and reach their goals and be fulfilled not only as athletes but also as well-rounded, successful individuals. It's these relationships that drive me every day when I wake up in the morning.

What we've been able to accomplish at Athletes' Performance is special, and I take great pride and responsibility in being able to share this with you. In fact, I'm so excited about this book that I want to make it possible for at least a few readers to come to Athletes' Performance and tell me their stories in person.

I want to hear about how *Core Performance* has transformed your life—and not just from a physical standpoint. Tell me how it's enabled you to meet challenges and fulfill your dreams. I want to hear about what you've overcome and the roadblocks you've navigated. Tell me how you've taken a more proactive approach to your life. (When you've gone through this program for 12 weeks, don't forget to go back and look at your answers in the self-evaluation. You'll be amazed at how your perspective has changed.)

Please share your stories with me at mark@coreperformance.com. We'll pick the most inspirational submissions, the ones that touch us the deepest, and bring the authors to Athletes' Performance to train in person with our staff, alongside some of the best athletes in the world. More important, I'll be able to meet you, and you can share with me personally how you transformed your life to accomplish your goals, motivating me even further.

I look forward to hearing from you.

Your coach,
Mark Verstegen

CHAPTER 16

FREQUENTLY ASKED QUESTIONS (FAQs)

Q: WILL I GAIN OR LOSE WEIGHT WITH THIS PROGRAM?

A: Don't get hung up on scale weight. If you step on a scale, it just gives you a number. It doesn't tell you how much muscle and fat you have. I can find two people the same height and weight that look dramatically different because of their body compositions.

People might weigh the same in their mid-forties as they did in their twenties, but they might have a lot more fat. Building lean mass is the key to success. To measure lean mass, perform the "pinch-an-inch" test by taking a vertical pinch of your skin by the navel. The thinner the pinch, the better.

We want to be less concerned with weight and more concerned with our ratio of lean mass to fat. With this program, you *should* expect to gain lean mass and lose fat. Remember, though, that a pound of lean mass takes up far less space than a pound of fat. If you're someone in reasonably good shape when you start this program, you could gain weight and look far leaner—or as some might say, "skinnier"—losing inches off your waistline. Most people would be surprised to know

that Nomar Garciaparra weighs 190 or that tennis player Meghann Shaughnessy weighs 150. By the standards of most people, they don't *look* that heavy. After all, Meghann wears size 4 clothes. But their ratios of lean mass to fat are exceptional.

If you're someone who begins this program overweight, you might not lose as much scale weight as you expect. But since you're reducing fat and increasing muscle, you'll look leaner and end up stronger than with traditional diet plans that promote weight loss, which is usually temporary, without building lean mass. There are NFL linemen who weigh 300 pounds when they arrive at Athletes' Performance, and after 3 months, they might weigh anywhere from 290 to 310, which by scale weight is an insignificant weight change for men of that size. But their ratio of lean mass to fat has tilted heavily in favor of lean mass; they've completely transformed their bodies.

Q: SHOULDN'T KIDS AVOID LIFTING WEIGHTS?

A: There's always been a school of thought that kids should avoid resistance training, since their bones are still growing. But look at how little kids move. They jump off a sliding board or climb monkey bars. They run down a basketball court or sprint across a field. There are more forces on joints and musculature in those movements than we could ever create with resistance training.

This workout is great for kids but, like anything else, there must be a level of mastery and progression. We're not going to hand a kid—or an adult—a huge weight without teaching him how to perform the movement properly with just his body weight. Once he's mastered that, we progress to a light weight. It's a progression, for kids as well as adults, that ensures safety throughout the Core Workout.

There is no chance that we're going to damage bones and stunt growth. This program will strengthen bones, improve posture, and lengthen and stabilize muscles. All of these will stimulate growth. Exercise causes the release of positive hormones. By eating properly, you're feeding your body so that it will reach its proper potential.

Kids should be able to do this program and feel as strong as they can, especially when it comes to pillar strength. When I think of the benefits this program will have, I'm incredibly excited for kids. This sports science wasn't around when I was growing up. If kids can start building pillar strength, think of the impact that will have on their long-term health, to say nothing of their competitive edge if they play sports.

Q: IT'S DIFFICULT TO REMEMBER PROPER FORM FOR SOME EXERCISES. WILL IT EVER BECOME SECOND NATURE?

A: Definitely. You're developing your body in such a way that you naturally hold these postures and go through these ranges of motion without thinking about them. We're reprogramming your "computer" so that you hold that perfect posture, that pillar strength, with the shoulder blades back and down, the belly button up and in, and the hips stabilized. If you can do that, you will do the majority of these exercises very well. Once we get those circuit breakers turned on and activated, they're on. It's like when you walk into the room and turn on the lights. They remain on; you don't have to keep holding the switch. After a while, you'll also bend properly without thinking about form. When we squat or bend, we need to do so from the hips *and* the knees, not at the waist. We need to sit the hips back and down, using the glutes and quads as opposed to just using the lower back or putting a lot of stress on our knees.

Q: AM I ALWAYS GOING TO FEEL SO UNBALANCED AND UNCOORDINATED?

A: No. Every athlete who comes to Athletes' Performance, regardless of skill level, feels awkward at first. It might take a few days or even a few weeks, but when you get it, it will change the way that your body works. Be patient; it's a new skill. If I was going to ask you to do only those things you're good at, you'd never improve. I want to push you beyond the limiting factors. Focus on the process, and the end result will come.

Q: WHY WON'T I GET BULKY DOING THIS PROGRAM?

A: Because there's the proper balance between the lengthening of the muscle and the stabilization of the muscle. The resistance training we're doing will take you through a long, full range of motion, which not only will help build muscle but also will improve the length of the muscle, so you have a long, lean, athletic look. And because you're gaining lean mass and losing fat, you'll avoid looking bulky since a pound of lean mass takes up far less space than a pound of fat.

Q: SHOULDN'T WE BE LIFTING WEIGHTS MORE OFTEN, ESPECIALLY EARLY ON?

A: You will be lifting quite often over the course of the 12-week program. Early on, I don't need you to do a lot of the same stuff. Instead, I want you to stabilize your body, elongate the muscles, and create muscle balance. I want you to concentrate on creating muscular balance and activating muscles properly. When you advance to more intense resistance training, you'll be much stronger and better balanced, even in exercises that you haven't attempted in a long time. In the first cycle, you might lift only a few times a week, but that

doesn't mean that you aren't doing resistive or strength training in other ways. Strength training is more than just lifting weights. It can be lifting your body, challenging the stabilizer muscles, or building elastic strength—all of which are necessary for a well-rounded program.

Q: I'M A DISTANCE RUNNER. WILL I BENEFIT FROM THIS PROGRAM?

A: Absolutely. This will significantly improve your endurance work, whether you're a runner, swimmer, or cyclist. Since you're already getting a lot of cardio work in, you could eliminate the Energy System Development (ESD) portion of this program, or you could apply it to your running, working in zones 1, 2, and 3.

Do, however, adapt your routine to the Core Workout. Since we work hard on Monday, Tuesday, Thursday, and Friday, you might want to do your long weekly run on Saturday. Or, if needed, you could alter your schedule to have two other pairs of back-to-back hard-training days—perhaps Tuesday/Wednesday, Friday/Saturday—with a long run on Sunday.

No matter how you break it down and adapt your routine, it will complement everything you're doing. You'll gain more distance on your strides because you're more flexible. The greater distance will make you faster. Every stride (or swim stroke or pedal revolution) will be more stable, allowing you to transfer energy more efficiently. By being more elastic, you'll efficiently store and release more energy with every stride, with less effort! And you'll efficiently increase your speed while decreasing your energy expenditure and level of effort at this pace, resulting in greater endurance and decreased times.

From just a regenerative standpoint, the AIS rope stretching, foam rolls, cold plunges, and Core Nutrition Plan will be a huge benefit. And by applying the same quality-over-quantity approach within the course of a workout and over a weekly schedule, you'll improve performance, even within your endurance workouts. That's how marathon runners learn to run at such a brisk pace. They first learn to run fast over short distances, then extend that pace over longer distances.

An endurance athlete on this program will have better results than she's had over any 12-week portion of her career.

Q: TO STAY THIN, I EAT FEW CARBOHYDRATES. AREN'T CARBS BAD FOR YOU?

A: Several popular diets advocate that you don't eat carbs, and that's one way to lose a lot of weight in a hurry. After all, for every gram of carbohydrate we eat, we store 3 grams of water. But that's a good thing since it keeps us hydrated and satiated.

If we go on one of those diets without carbs, it's like taking a sponge and wringing the water out. You'll lose the water weight, but as soon as you eat carbs again—and you will at some point because you need energy and can only go so long without carbs—then that sponge is going to fill up with water. When it does, that weight is going to come right back. Not only that, but a low-carb diet is going to leave your body deficient in many vitamins and minerals and lacking in fiber.

Q: HOW MANY SHAKES DO I NEED A DAY?

A: That depends on your lifestyle. With this program, you need a minimum of one, taken immediately following your workout or as a preworkout shooter. Either way, you'll maximize the recovery process. If your lifestyle makes it more convenient to have a high-protein meal-replacement bar or shake in the afternoon and/or late evening, by all means do so. The important thing is to eat often, five or six times a day. By no means, however, must you drink two or more shakes a day.

Q: CAN I DO THIS PROGRAM IF I HAVE ARTHRITIS?

A: It depends. For some people, arthritis is self-diagnosed because they have joint pain, which comes from dysfunction because of imbalance and tightness in muscles. That changes the function of a joint and creates more pain. When that happens, you shut those muscles down even more, and it perpetuates the problem further.

Throughout this program, you're going to change the tissue so that it's more pliable. By doing Movement Prep and AIS rope stretching and using the foam roll, you're taking dry, brittle, stiff tissue and lubricating it so that the muscles and joints function again. You're going to change the muscle by elongating the tissue, breaking up the adhesions, turning on and re-programming the nervous system, and creating muscular balance. That way, the joint will be in a happy environment and function properly, reversing this degrading process and improving the quality of your life.

Q: WHAT ABOUT ALCOHOL?

A: We're trying to build this program around your lifestyle. I'm not going to tell you to abstain from everything; if I do, you won't comply with the program. Alcohol may be a part of your lifestyle, but I ask you to minimize it, maybe to one or two drinks per week. If you're going to have more than that, then I hope you'll have drinks with some health benefit, such as red wines, which have flavonoids that act as antioxidants. Always drink one glass of water for every alcoholic drink.

Q: HOW ABOUT SMOKING?

A: This might be a strange question to bring up, but I'm amazed how many smokers spend hours in the gym without addressing this obvious problem. Smoking raises metabolism and kills your tastebuds so you eat less, but it's a terrible way to stay thin.

If you look at the function of your body and your ability to maintain health and quality of life for as long as possible, the last thing you'd want to do is put your mouth around an exhaust pipe, and then do this multiple times a day for years on end. If you're going to make this commitment to the Core Workout and adopt all these new philosophies and programs, this is the time to turn over a new leaf and kick that bad habit. Let that nicotine drop and replace it with the natural endorphin high that you'll get from this program.

Q: HOW MUCH WATER SHOULD I DRINK?

A: You cannot drink too much. Drink as much as you physically can. If you increase your hydration status, the worst thing that's going to happen is that you'll sweat it out or pee it out. If you're not hydrated enough, you're going to have a false sense of appetite and limited ability to perform your workouts.

So drink water. It'll help with your flexibility, strength, and well-being, and it helps all of your internal components with flushing out your system. I recommend drinking 64 to 96 ounces of water a day. If that seems impossible, add up all the ounces of soft drinks, diet cola, and coffee you consume a day. I'm not necessarily asking you to drink more liquid—just replace your existing drinks with water.

Q: WHAT ABOUT SPORTS DRINKS?

A: Some are better than others, and all are engineered to contain higher glycemic carbohydrates, sodium, and electrolytes, which are best utilized during intense or strenuous activity. If you're inactive, or slightly active, and are drinking a lot of sugary beverages, you'll have continually elevated levels of blood sugar, which exceed your needs and may be stored as fat.

If you plan to utilize sports drinks, make sure to use them at appropriate times; otherwise, drink water or try some of the new "fitness waters," such as Gatorade Propel, for some added taste.

Q: IF NUTS HAVE A HIGH PERCENTAGE OF FAT, AREN'T THEY BAD FOR YOU?

A: Nuts provide good, unsaturated fats and are a good source of protein and fiber. A handful of nuts is a healthy, low-glycemic snack. Nuts also can be a nutritious topping for salads and dishes.

Q: I TRAVEL A LOT FOR BUSINESS. HOW CAN I EVER KEEP UP WITH THIS?

A: I travel a lot. So do many of our athletes. Admittedly, there might be times when we don't have as much equipment as we'd like, although physioballs and cable-lifting machines have become common in hotel gyms. Like anything else, it's important to plan ahead. Pack a rope for your AIS stretching. Throw some high-protein meal-replacement bars and packets of postworkout recovery mix in your bag so that you don't have to resort to junk food.

If it gets to be the end of the day and you've found you haven't exercised, do something in your hotel room. Go through the Movement Prep routine. Work on some of the core/hip/shoulder stability routines. Take out the rope. It's especially important to work out when you're traveling because of all the stress traveling puts on you. You're inevitably stiff and cramped from sitting in a tiny airline seat. Your body might be trying to adjust to a new time zone. Do what you can to keep from getting run-down.

The worst thing about traveling is being away from family, but if there is a silver lining, it's that you might have a little more time early in the morning and in the evening to work out—even if it's an abbreviated version of the Core Workout (see page 198).

Q: WHAT DO I DO WHEN I'VE COMPLETED PHASE 4 AFTER 12 WEEKS?

A: For starters, take that week or long weekend you scheduled and "reload." Go on vacation or at least do something near home that you enjoy. Once you return, go back to the extensive phase (phase 2) and repeat the last three phases at a much higher level. Increase the weight. Go for more reps. Perfect your form. You'll find you can do the workout much more quickly.

Once you've accomplished that, log on to our Web site, www.coreperformance.com, for some advanced training techniques that build upon what you've already mastered. That way you can customize this program to your own needs and experience.

Q: IF I HAVE ONLY 30 MINUTES TO WORK OUT, SHOULD I LIFT WEIGHTS OR DO CARDIO WORK?

A: Neither. I want you to change your mindset and think about the maximum possible total-body result in that time frame.

I'd want you to do the Movement Prep unit and some combination of our Strength unit (which obviously involves lifting weights) and the Elasticity unit. That way, you'll get mobility and stability work, along with a strength workout. You'll burn calories by going through these units rapidly, which will be equivalent to Energy System Development (ESD) work. Plus you'll get the long-term benefit of having your body use calories to repair and improve your lean body mass.

Q: WON'T WOMEN GET BULKY IN THIS PROGRAM?

A: No. Whether you're male or female, I don't want you to become bulky. I want you to be long and lean, which is to say that you will have elongated muscles and decreased body fat. You will have lean body mass and be able to see muscles.

Q: I WORK OUT ALL THE TIME. HOW COME I DON'T SEE THE RESULTS?

A: Chances are, you have only part of the formula. Perhaps you're not undergoing any type of Regeneration and are therefore not letting the body recover from stress. Or maybe you have been doing the same workout for so long, your body has grown accustomed to it. Perhaps you're not following a proper nutrition plan. *Core Performance* is a complete, integrated plan that will continually challenge you.

Q: DO YOU RECOMMEND ANY SUPPLEMENTS BEYOND THOSE THAT ARE LISTED IN THE TEXT?

A: We've tried to keep things simple with the preworkout shooter or postworkout recovery mix, antioxidant complex, and multivitamin. Beyond that, you might want to consider a digestive enzyme complex, which helps the body get the most out of foods. Take that with every meal. You could add some vitamin C for its antioxidant properties and take it early in the morning or in the evening. A bottle of joint-support formula promotes healthy joints, if you think you need help in that area.

Q: WHAT ABOUT CREATINE?

A: If you're maximizing all the other benefits of *Core Performance,* you might want to consider adding creatine after the first 6 to 12 weeks of the program. Creatine, which is produced in the body and found in meat and fish, helps the muscles recover between sets and helps you develop explosive strength. It is similar to a carbohydrate in that it is stored in the muscles and its level fluctuates. It's most effective to take creatine in 3-week cycles, alternating between 3 weeks of taking it and 3 weeks without. Take 5 to 10 grams of creatine per day, ideally first thing in the morning on an empty stomach. If you work out in the morning, you could add it to your preworkout shooter.

Q: I DO PILATES OR YOGA. SHOULD I CONTINUE TO DO SO?

A: Absolutely. We've incorporated elements of Pilates and yoga, along with dance and martial arts, into our programs. I'd recommend doing Pilates or yoga on your recovery days in place of Prehab or the Physioball Routine.

GLOSSARY OF TERMS

Abductors: The outer-thigh muscles located on the sides of your hips. They are important for lateral movement and stabilization.

Active rest: Time off from regular training. The *active* refers to hobbies or sports that involve some degree of physical activity.

Adductors: The muscles located in your inner thigh. They help pull your legs back toward your body and stabilize your hips and pelvis.

Amino acids: The main material of the body's cells. They're the building blocks from which proteins and muscle are made.

Antioxidants: Chemical compounds that neutralize the cellular-damaging effects of free radicals. Antioxidants slow the aging process, ward off cancer and stress, and promote good health.

Athletic position: The proper form for sport-related movement. Hold perfect posture (shoulder blades back and down and tummy tight). Keep your legs slightly bent with your hips sitting back and down. Your weight should be forward, on the middle of your feet.

Body composition: The percentage of body weight composed of fat as opposed to lean mass (usually expressed in terms of a body-fat percentage—12 percent, for example, which is typical for a male team-sport athlete). "Body comp" is a more accurate barometer of overall fitness than "scale weight."

Calorie: The unit to measure energy that comes from food.

Carbohydrate: Along with protein and fat, one of the three main classifications of foods (macronutrients). A main source of energy for the body, "carbs" are mostly sugars and starches that the body breaks down to the simple sugar glucose to feed its cells. There are, on average, 4 calories per gram of carbohydrate.

Cholesterol: A fatlike substance found in blood, muscle, brain, and other tissue, it's a vital component in the production of many hormones. Too much cholesterol can cause fat to build up in arteries and lead to heart disease and stroke.

Concentric: The lifting portion of a resistance exercise, when the muscle shortens or contracts. With the bench press, for instance, the concentric phase occurs when you press the weight from your chest back up to the starting position.

Eccentric: The lowering portion of a resistance exercise, when the muscle lengthens. With the bench press, the eccentric phase occurs when you lower the bar from the starting position to your chest.

Fascia: Connective tissue that envelops the muscles, interacts with joints, and attaches to bones. Fascia holds the body together and gives it structure and shape. Fascia organizes and separates, providing protection and autonomy for individual muscles.

Fat: Along with carbohydrate and protein, one of the three main classifications of foods (macronutrients). Fats serve as energy stores for the body and have antioxidant properties. In food, there are two types of fat: unsaturated (good) and saturated (bad). A gram of fat contains 9 calories.

Fructose: Sugar that is found in fruits and vegetables.

Glucose: Also known as dextrose, a simple sugar found in the blood that serves as the body's main source of energy.

Glutes: A group of muscles also known as the rear hips or butt.

Glycemic index: A measure of a single food's effect on blood sugar levels over time. Foods with a higher glycemic response quickly raise blood sugar levels, resulting in wild fluctuations in energy level and mood.

Glycemic load: A measure of a food's portion size on blood sugar levels over time. The glycemic load is computed by taking the food's glycemic index and multiplying it by the number of calories. The exact formula is (glycemic index $\times$ .01) multiplied by the number of calories per serving.

Glycemic response: The cumulative effect of all foods eaten at one time on the body's blood sugar level over time.

Glycogen: The most immediately available source of stored fuel in the body. Made up of sugars and stored in the liver and muscles, it releases glucose when needed by the cells.

Grazing: The philosophy of eating smaller meals throughout the day as opposed to three heavy, sit-down affairs.

High-fructose corn syrup (HFCS): A highly processed sweetener that was popularized in the 1970s by food manufacturers looking for a cheap substitute for cane sugar. Found in many everyday foods such as soft drinks, condiments, and breads, HFCS sends blood sugar levels sky-high before they crash quickly, making the body hungry for even more high-glycemic food.

Hot/cold contrasts (plunging): The process of immersing the body in alternating temperature extremes to increase blood flow and promote muscle recovery. Most commonly done in hot tubs/cold plunges, baths, or the shower.

Iliotibial (IT) band: A thick band of tissue on the side of your leg that extends from the thigh down over the knee and attaches to the tibia (shinbone).

Isometric: A contraction in which there is no change in muscle length. For example, when you lift a dumbbell to a particular height and hold it there, the muscle is in isometric contraction.

Lactate threshold: The point in working out where the demand for cellular energy (lactate) equals the supply. If athletes can raise their lactate thresholds, they will be able to perform high-intensity work for longer periods.

Omega-3 fatty acids: Found in flaxseed oil, fish oils, and cold-water fish, these are an essential part of the diet and believed to reduce risk of cardiovascular disease.

Overtraining: When the effect of working out exceeds the body's ability to recover. Common symptoms of overtraining include sleep disturbances, joint pain, headaches, poor appetite, and lowered resistance to illness (more colds and sinus infections, for example).

Perfect posture: The proper stance for optimal movement. Shoulder blades should be pulled back and down, and the tummy should be drawn up and in, activating the transverse abdominis. There should be a straight line from the ears to the shoulders, the shoulders to the hips, the hips to the knees, and the knees to the ankles.

Physioball: Also known as a stability, balance, or Swiss ball, a large rubber inflatable ball used to challenge the body to build greater stability and proprioception.

Pillar (strength): The torso and associated elements (core, hip, and shoulder stability and strength) that form the foundation for all movement, providing a center axis from which to move. If the body is a wheel, the pillar is the hub and the limbs the spokes.

Postworkout recovery mix: A protein-rich powder that's combined with water or juice to make a liquid meal that accelerates workout recovery, builds lean body mass, and accounts for 40 to 100 percent of the daily recommended allowance of 25 vitamins and minerals per serving.

Prehabilitation (prehab): The proactive means of training and conditioning often-injured areas of the body, such as the shoulders and hips, to prevent injuries and surgeries that would require rehabilitation, or rehab.

Preworkout shooter: A glass of water or diluted fruit juice mixed with a scoop of whey protein and consumed before a workout to give the body a head start on postworkout muscle recovery.

Prone: Lying on the stomach with the face down.

Proprioception: The system of pressure sensors in the joints, muscles, and tendons, which provide the body with information to maintain balance.

Protein: Along with carbohydrate and fat, one of the three main classifications of food (macronutrients). Proteins are made of amino acids, the building blocks of lean body mass. Cells need protein for growth and repair. The body breaks down protein to produce amino acids. Protein is found in many foods such as fish, meat, poultry, eggs, and dairy products.

There are 4 calories in a gram of protein, on average.

Reciprocal inhibition: The neuromuscular response between opposing muscle groups, especially in relation to how they interact, with one relaxing when the other one fires.

Recovery: A low-intensity training unit to help the body repair itself following more intense training.

Regeneration: Nutritional supplements and planned activities to help the body physically or psychologically overcome the stress of training.

Satiety: The state of feeling full and satisfied after eating, as opposed to hungry.

Saturated fats: These are "bad" fats since they tend to raise blood cholesterol. Saturated fats are solid at room temperature and come mainly from animal food products such as butter, lard, and meat fat.

Scapula: Either of a pair of large, flat triangular bones that form the back part of the shoulder and serve as the foundation for all arm movement.

Seamless integration: The notion of weaving various disciplines and philosophies into one training and lifestyle program for maximum benefit, as opposed to the traditional training philosophy of working body parts.

Skinny fat: Refers to a thin person who has a high ratio of fat to lean mass, almost always because of a poor nutritional program.

Supine: Lying on the back with the face up.

Trans fat: An artery-clogging fat formed during hydrogenation, which converts liquid oil to a solid fat. Found in processed foods such as cookies, crackers, and margarine, trans fat raises bad cholesterol (LDL) but doesn't raise good (HDL) cholesterol.

Transverse abdominis (TA): A remarkable sheath of muscle that originates from the spine and wraps around and attaches to the torso and pelvis, serving as nature's "weight belt." The transverse abdominis is the first muscle to fire in all movement.

Unsaturated fat: These are usually "good" fats, since they don't raise blood cholesterol. Unsaturated fats, which include monounsaturated and polyunsaturated fats, are liquid at room temperature and come from oils such as fish, flaxseed, olive, and canola.

Whey protein: A powerful protein (pronounced "way") that includes many essential amino acids that boost the immune system and promote overall good health.

ADDITIONAL TRAINING LOGS

An important goal of *Core Performance* is getting you more excited about exercise, about developing elements of fitness and athleticism that go beyond the one-dimensional benefits of bodybuilding, endurance training, yoga, or anything else you've tried.

And, after 12 weeks of the Core Workout, I hope I've succeeded.

That brings up the inevitable question: What's next?

First, of course, I hope you'll take a week off from serious exercise to allow your body to fully recover and to help heal any nagging aches or pains that may have cropped up. (Believe me, they happen to everybody.)

Second, reconsider your goals and plan to refocus your workout around them. If you want to add more muscle size, that means using heavier weights, doing fewer repetitions, and taking more rest between sets. If you're aiming for more fat loss, you might consider adding some sets, with less rest in between.

Whatever those goals turn out to be, you can easily achieve them by repeating the Core Workout (starting with Phase 2, since your body doesn't need another break-in phase) and making those adjustments. You'll find new training logs on the following pages, and you're welcome to make any adjustments to the program that you wish. Swap out some of my exercises for some of your own. (You'll find plenty of new workout ideas at www.coreperformance.com.) Add sets, change repetition schemes—whatever you think will push you closer to your goals.

I just want you to remember to incorporate all of the Super Seven—Movement Prep, Prehab, Physioball Routine, Elasticity, Strength, Energy System Development, and Regeneration. That's why you'll find the program printed in full on the following pages. I hope you'll photocopy those pages, make your changes, follow that routine to completion, then come back and create another program based on this configuration and these principles.

THE CORE WORKOUT

Phase 2: Extensive (Weeks 4, 5, and 6)
Goals: Increase elasticity, strength, work capacity/quantity

MONDAY	TUESDAY	WEDNESDAY
Movement Prep A&B (12 min.)	Movement Prep A (6 min.)	ESD 3 (30 min.)
Prehab: Core (7 min.)	Strength A (25 min.)	Physioball (12 min.)
Prehab: Hip (7 min.)	ESD 4 (15 min.)	**Total Time: 42 min.**
Prehab: Shoulder (7 min.)	**Total Time: 46 min.**	Regeneration: Foam (6 min.)
Elasticity (10 min.)		Regeneration: AIS (12 min.)
Total Time: 43 min.		
Regeneration: Foam (7 min.)		

STRENGTH: 30-Second Rest between Sets

TEMPO: 311

STRENGTH A		Tuesday	Tuesday	Tuesday
SUPERSET				
Bench Press	set 1	8	8	8
	set 2	8	8	6
	set 3	8	6	6
Romanian Deadlift (RDL)	set 1	8	8	8
	set 2	8	8	6
	set 3	8	6	6
SUPERSET				
Split Squat/Lunge	set 1	8@	8@	8@
	set 2	8@	8@	6@
	set 3	8@	8@	6@
Pullup (horiz. to vert.)	set 1	6	8	10
	set 2	6	8	10
	set 3	6	8	10
CIRCUIT				
Cable 1-Arm Rot. Row	set 1	8@	8@	8@
	set 2	8@	8@	8@
Split DB Curl-to-Press	set 1	5@	5@	5@
	set 2	4@	4@	4@
DB Pullover Extension	set 1	10	10	10
	set 2	8	8	8

	THURSDAY	FRIDAY	SATURDAY
	Movement Prep A&B (12 min.)	Movement Prep B (6 min.)	ESD 3 (30 min.)
	Prehab: Core (7 min.)	Strength B (20 min.)	Physioball (12 min.)
	Prehab: Hip (7 min.)	ESD 5 (15 min.)	**Total Time: 42 min.**
	Prehab: Shoulder (7 min.)	**Total Time: 41 min.**	Regeneration: Foam (5+ min.)
	Elasticity (10 min.)		Regeneration: AIS (5+ min.)
	Total Time: 43 min.		
	Regeneration: Foam (7 min.)		

Full Range of Motion and Adhere to 311 Tempo!

STRENGTH B			Friday	Friday	Friday
SUPERSET					
Alt DB Bench Press	set 1		10	10	8
	set 2		10	8	8
Split Squat/Lunge	set 1		10@	10@	8@
	set 2		10@	10@	8@
SUPERSET					
1-Arm, 1-Leg DB Row	set 1		10@	10@	8@
	set 2		10@	10@	8@
Floor/PB Leg Curl	set 1		8	10	12
	set 2		8	10	12
CIRCUIT					
Cable Lifting	set 1		10@	10@	10@
	set 2		8@	8@	8@
Cable Chopping	set 1		10@	10@	10@
	set 2		8@	8@	8@
Split DB Curl-to-Press	set 1		5@	5@	5@
	set 2		4@	4@	4@

THE CORE WORKOUT (CONT.)

Phase 2: Extensive (Weeks 4, 5, and 6)
Goals: Increase elasticity, strength, work capacity/quantity

MOVEMENT PREP

MOVEMENT PREP A	Week 1	Week 2	Week 3
Forward Lunge/Forearm-to-Instep	1 × 5@	1 × 6@	1 × 7@
Backward Lunge with a Twist	1 × 5@	1 × 6@	1 × 7@
Calf Stretch	1 × 10@	1 × 12@	1 × 7@
Hand Walk	1 × 5	1 × 6	1 × 7
Inverted Hamstring	1 × 5@	1 × 6@	1 × 7@

MOVEMENT PREP B	Week 1	Week 2	Week 3
Hip Crossover	1 × 10@ to 90° knees	1 × 12@ to longer legs	1 × 7@ to ¾ to straight legs
Scorpion	1 × 10@	1 × 12@	1 × 7@
Lateral Lunge	1 × 5@	1 × 6@	1 × 7@
Drop Lunge	1 × 5@	1 × 6@	1 × 7@
Sumo Squat-to-Stand	1 × 5	1 × 6	1 × 7

PREHAB

PREHAB: SHOULDER	Week 1	Week 2	Week 3
Floor/PB *T*	1 × 8 + weight	1 × 10 + weight	1 × 12 + weight
Floor/PB *W*	1 × 8 + weight	1 × 10 + weight	1 × 12 + weight
Floor/PB *L*	1 × 8 + weight	1 × 10 + weight	1 × 12 + weight
PB Pushup Plus	1 × 8	1 × 10	1 × 12
PB Reach, Roll, and Lift	1 × 10	1 × 12	1 × 14

PREHAB: HIP	Week 1	Week 2	Week 3
Glute Bridge with Adduction	1 × 10	1 × 12	1 × 14
Side-Lying Ad/Abduction	1 × 10@	1 × 12@	1 × 14@
Quadruped Circles	1 × 5@	1 × 6@	1 × 7@

PREHAB: CORE	Week 1	Week 2	Week 3
Pillar Bridge Front	1 × 30 sec.	1 × 45 sec.	1 × 60 sec.
Pillar Bridge Side (right/left)	1 × 30 sec.@	1 × 45 sec.@	1 × 60 sec.@

ELASTICITY

Exercise	Week 1	Week 2	Week 3
Base Side-to-Side (fast)	2 × 6 sec.	2 × 8 sec.	2 × 10 sec.
Base Rotation (fast)	2 × 6 sec.	2 × 8 sec.	2 × 10 sec.
Squat Jump	2 × 5 reps	2 × 6 reps	2 × 7 reps
Lateral Bound	2 × 3 reps@	2 × 4 reps@	2 × 4 reps@

PHYSIOBALL

Exercise	Week 1	Week 2	Week 3
Lateral Roll	1 × 10@	1 × 12@	1 × 14@
Russian Twist	1 × 10 add weight@	1 × 12 + more weight@	1 × 14 + more weight@
Plate Crunch	1 × 10 add weight	1 × 12 + more weight	1 × 14 + more weight
Knee Tuck	1 × 10	1 × 12	1 × 14
Lying Opposites	1 × 10@	1 × 12@	1 × 14@
Reverse Hyper	1 × 10	1 × 12	1 × 14
Reverse Crunch	1 × 10	1 × 12	1 × 14
Bridging	1 × 10	1 × 12	1 × 14
Hip Crossover	1 × 10@	1 × 12@	1 × 14@

ESD

Workout	Total/# Reps	Warmup	Work/Zone	Rest/Zone
4 Lactate Capacity	15 min./3 reps	3 min./Z1	2 min./Z2	2 min./Z1
5 Lactate Capacity	15 min./2 reps	3 min./Z1	3 min./Z2	3 min./Z1
3 Aerobic/Recovery	—	—	30+ min./Z1	—

REGENERATION

Exercise	Week 1	Week 2	Week 3
Foam Hamstring	1 × 8@	1 × 10@	1 × 12@
Foam IT Band	1 × 8@	1 × 10@	1 × 12@
Foam Quad	1 × 8@	1 × 10@	1 × 12@
Foam Glute	1 × 8	1 × 10	1 × 12
Foam Back	1 × 8	1 × 10	1 × 12
AIS Rope Calf	1 × 8@	1 × 10@	1 × 12@
AIS Rope Hamstring	1 × 8@	1 × 10@	1 × 12@
AIS Rope IT/Glute	1 × 8@	1 × 10@	1 × 12@
AIS Rope Adductors	1 × 8@	1 × 10@	1 × 12@
AIS Rope Quad/Hip	1 × 8@	1 × 10@	1 × 12@
AIS Rope Chest	1 × 8	1 × 10	1 × 12
AIS Rope Triceps	1 × 8@	1 × 10@	1 × 12@
AIS 90/90 Stretch	1 × 8@	1 × 10@	1 × 12@
AIS Quadruped Rocking	1 × 8	1 × 10	1 × 12

If you're pressed for time, select the 4 AIS stretches that best target your problem areas.

THE CORE WORKOUT

Phase 3: Intensive (Weeks 7, 8, and 9)
Intermediate/Advanced
Goals: Speed, Power, Strength, Quality

MONDAY	TUESDAY	WEDNESDAY
Movement Prep A (6 min.)	Movement Prep B (5 min.)	ESD 3 (30 min.)
Elasticity A (10 min.)	Elasticity B (10 min.)	Prehab: Core (10 min.)
Strength A (30 min.)	Strength B (30 min.)	**Total Time: 40 min.**
Prehab: Shoulder (5 min.)	ESD 8 (15 min.)	Nutrition: Shake
Total Time: 51 min.	**Total Time: 60 min.**	Regeneration: Foam (10 min.)
Nutrition: Shake	Nutrition: Shake	Regeneration: AIS (10 min.)

STRENGTH: 60-Second Rest between Supersets   TEMPO: 30X (Explosive)

STRENGTH A		Monday	Thursday	Monday	Thursday	Monday	Thursday
SUPERSET							
Bench Press+Plyo Pushup	set 1	5+3*	8+3*	4+3*	8+3*	3+3*	6
	set 2	5+3*	8+3*	4+3*	8+3*	3+3*	**
	set 3	5+3*	8+3*	4+3*	8+3*	3+3*	**
Pullup (add weight)	set 1	6	6	4	4	3	6
	set 2	6	6	4	4	3	**
	set 3	6	6	4	4	3	**
SUPERSET							
DB Pullover Extension	set 1	6	8	5	8	4	6
	set 2	6	8	5	8	4	**
DB Curl-to-Press	set 1	6	8	5	8	4	6
	set 2	6	8	5	8	4	**
SUPERSET							
Cable Chopping	set 1	8@	8@	6@	6@	6@	6@
	set 2	8@	8@	6@	6@	6@	6@
Cable Lifting	set 1	8@	8@	6@	6@	6@	6@
	set 2	8@	8@	6@	6@	6@	6@

*Do 3 plyo pushups after each bench press set, then rest 60 seconds, do pullups, then rest 60 seconds and repeat.

**Do maximum reps with whatever weight you used in the first workout of this phase.

		THURSDAY	FRIDAY	SATURDAY

THURSDAY
Movement Prep A (6 min.)
Elasticity A (10 min.)
Strength A (30 min.)
Prehab: Shoulder (5 min.)
Total Time: 51 min.
Nutrition: Shake
Regeneration: Foam (7 min.)

FRIDAY
Movement Prep B (5 min.)
Elasticity B (10 min.)
Strength B (30 min.)
ESD 9 (17 min.)
Total Time: 62 min.
Nutrition: Shake

SATURDAY
ESD 3 (30 min.)
Prehab: Core (10 min.)
Total Time: 40 min.
Nutrition: Shake
Regeneration: Foam (10 min.)
Regeneration: AIS (10 min.)

Full Range of Motion and Adhere to 30X Tempo!

STRENGTH B		Tuesday	Friday	Tuesday	Friday	Tuesday	Friday
SUPERSET							Reload—Do Wednesday workout
Cable 1-Arm Rot. Row	set 1	8@	8@	6@	6@	6@	
	set 2	8@	8@	6@	6@	6@	
PB Russian Twist with weight	set 1	12@	12@	10@	10@	8@	
	set 2	12@	12@	10@	10@	8@	
SUPERSET							
Split Squat+Split Jump	set 1	6+3*	6+3*	4+3*	4+3*	3+3*	
	set 2	6+3*	6+3*	4+3*	4+3*	3+3*	
PB Plate Crunch	set 1	12	12	10	10	8	
	set 2	12	12	10	10	8	
SUPERSET							
DB Front Squat+Press+Squat Jump	set 1	8+4**	8+4**	6+4**	6+4**	4+4**	
	set 2	8+4**	8+4**	6+4**	6+4**	4+4**	
PB Lateral Roll	set 1	12@	12@	10@	10@	8@	
	set 2	12@	12@	10@	10@	8@	
SUPERSET							
Romanian Deadlift (RDL)	set 1	8	6	6	6	6	
	set 2	8	6	6	6	6	
PB Prone Knee Tuck	set 1	8	8	10	10	12	
	set 2	8	8	10	10	12	

*Do 3 split jumps after each set of 6 split squat lunges, then immediately do PB plate crunches.
** Do 4 squat jumps after each set of 8 DB front squat/presses, then immediately do PB lateral rolls.

THE CORE WORKOUT (CONT.)

Phase 3: Intensive (Weeks 7, 8, and 9)
Intermediate/Advanced
Goals: Speed, Power, Strength, Quality

MOVEMENT PREP

MOVEMENT PREP A	Week 1	Week 2	Week 3
Forward Lunge/Forearm-to-Instep	1 × 5@	1 × 6@	1 × 7@
Backward Lunge with a Twist	1 × 5@	1 × 6@	1 × 7@
Calf Stretch	1 × 10@	1 × 12@	1 × 14@
Hand Walk	1 × 5	1 × 6	1 × 7
Inverted Hamstring	1 × 5@	1 × 6@	1 × 7@
MOVEMENT PREP B	Week 1	Week 2	Week 3
Hip Crossover	1 × 10@ to 90° knees	1 × 12@ to longer legs	1 × 14@ to straight legs
Scorpion	1 × 10@	1 × 12@	1 × 14@
Lateral Lunge	1 × 5@	1 × 6@	1 × 14@
Drop Lunge	1 × 5@	1 × 6@	1 × 14@
Sumo Squat-to-Stand	1 × 5	1 × 6	1 × 7
Prehab Hip: Glute Bridge (1 leg)	1 × 10@	1 × 12@	1 × 14@

PREHAB

PREHAB: SHOULDER	Week 1	Week 2	Week 3
PB *Y*	1 × 10 + weight	1 × 12 + weight	1 × 12 + weight
PB *T*	1 × 10 + weight	1 × 12 + weight	1 × 12 + weight
PB *W*	1 × 10 + weight	1 × 12 + weight	1 × 12 + weight
PB *L*	1 × 10 + weight	1 × 12 + weight	1 × 12 + weight
PREHAB: CORE	Week 1	Week 2	Week 3
Pillar Bridge Front	2 × 20 sec.	2 × 30 sec.	2 × 40 sec.
Pillar Bridge Side (right/left) Top Leg	2 × 20 sec.	2 × 30 sec.	2 × 40 sec.
Pillar Bridge Side (right/left) Bottom Leg	2 × 20 sec.	2 × 30 sec.	2 × 40 sec.

ELASTICITY

ELASTICITY A	Week 1	Week 2	Week 3
1 Leg over the Line	2 × 5 sec.	2 × 7 sec.	2 × 7 sec.
Get-Up	4 reps	5 reps	6 reps
Side-to-Side Jump-to-Sprint	2 × 4 jumps each side	3 × 5 jumps each side	4 × 6 jumps each side

ELASTICITY B	Week 1	Week 2	Week 3
Lateral Bound	2 × 5@	2 × 6@	2 × 7@
3-Hurdle Drill	3 × 8 sec.	4 × 8 sec.	4 × 10 sec.

ESD

Workout	Total/# Reps	Warmup	Work/Zone	Rest/Zone
8 Lactate Power	15 min./4 reps/2 sets	3 min./Z1	30 sec./Z3	1 min./Z1
9 Lactate Power	15 min./4 reps	3 min./Z1	1 min./Z3	2 min./Z1
3 Aerobic/Recovery	—	—	30+ min./Z1	—

REGENERATION (Done Anytime/Anywhere!)

Exercise	Week 1	Week 2	Week 3
Foam Hamstring	1 × 8@	1 × 10@	1 × 12@
Foam IT Band	1 × 8@	1 × 10@	1 × 12@
Foam Quad/Groin	1 × 8@	1 × 10@	1 × 12@
Foam Glute	1 × 8	1 × 10	1 × 12
Foam Back/Lat	1 × 8@	1 × 10@	1 × 12@
AIS Rope Calf	1 × 8@	1 × 10@	1 × 12@
AIS Rope Hamstring	1 × 8@	1 × 10@	1 × 12@
AIS Rope or Static IT/Glute	1 × 8@	1 × 10@	1 × 12@
AIS Rope Adductors	1 × 8@	1 × 10@	1 × 12@
AIS Rope or Static Quad/Hip	1 × 8@	1 × 10@	1 × 12@
AIS Shoulder (Side-Lying)	1 × 8@	1 × 10@	1 × 12@
AIS Rope Triceps	1 × 8@	1 × 10@	1 × 12@
AIS 90/90 Stretch	1 × 8@	1 × 10@	1 × 12@
AIS Quadruped Rocking	1 × 8	1 × 10	1 × 12

If you're pressed for time, select the 4 AIS stretches that best target your problem areas.

THE CORE WORKOUT

Phase 4: Mixed (Weeks 10, 11, and 12—Week 13 Reload!)
Goals: Speed, Power, Strength, Quality

<table>
<tr><td>MONDAY
Movement Prep A (6 min.)
Elasticity A (10 min.)
Prehab: Shoulder (5 min.)
Strength A (25 min.)
ESD 10 (11 min.)
Total Time: 57 min.</td><td>TUESDAY
Movement Prep B (6 min.)
Elasticity B (10 min.)
Strength B (30 min.)
ESD 11 (15 min.)
Total Time: 61 min.</td><td>WEDNESDAY
ESD 3 (30 min.)
Prehab: Core (5 min.)
Regeneration: Foam (8 min.)
Regeneration: AIS (10 min.)
Total Time: 53 min.</td></tr>
</table>

STRENGTH: 30-Second Rest between Supersets   TEMPO: 30X (Explosive)

STRENGTH A		Monday	Thursday	Monday	Thursday	Monday	Thursday
SUPERSET							
Bench Press+PB Pushup	set 1	6+5	8+5	6+5	8+5	6+5	8+5
	set 2	4+5	6+5	4+5	6+5	4+5	6+5
	set 3	2+5	4+5	2+5	4+5	2+5	4+5
Split Squat+Split Jump	set 1	6+3	8+3	6+3	8+3	6+3	8+3
	set 2	4+3	6+3	4+3	6+3	4+3	6+3
	set 3	2+3	4+3	2+3	4+3	2+3	4+3
SUPERSET							
Kneeling/Cable Lifting	set 1	6@	8@	5@	7@	4@	6@
	set 2	6@	8@	5@	7@	4@	6@
Front Squat-to-Press	set 1	6	8	5	7	4	6
	set 2	6	8	5	7	4	6
DB Pullover Extension	set 1	10	10	8	8	6	6
	set 2	10	10	8	8	6	6

<table>
<tr><td colspan="2">THURSDAY</td><td colspan="2">FRIDAY</td><td colspan="2">SATURDAY</td></tr>
</table>

THURSDAY
Movement Prep A (6 min.)
Elasticity A (10 min.)
Prehab: Shoulder (5 min.)
Strength A (25 min.)
ESD 10 (11 min.)
Total Time: 57 min.

FRIDAY
Movement Prep B (6 min.)
Elasticity B (10 min.)
Strength B (30 min.)
ESD 11 (15 min.)
Total Time: 61 min.

SATURDAY
ESD 3 (30 min.)
Prehab: Core (5 min.)
Regeneration: Foam (8 min.)
Regeneration: AIS (10 min.)
Total Time: 53 min.

Full Range of Motion and Adhere to 30X Tempo!

STRENGTH B		Tuesday	Friday	Tuesday	Friday	Tuesday	Friday
SUPERSET							
Cable 1-Arm Rot. Row	set 1	8@	8@	6@	6@	6@	6@
	set 2	8@	8@	6@	6@	6@	6@
PB Russian Twist	set 1	12	12	15	15	18	18
	set 2	12	12	15	15	18	18
SUPERSET							
1-Arm, 1-Leg DB Row	set 1	6@	8@	5@	7@	4@	6@
	set 2	6@	8@	5@	7@	4@	6@
PB Prone Knee Tuck (1 leg)	set 1	8@	8@	10@	10@	12@	12@
	set 2	8@	8@	10@	10@	12@	12@
SUPERSET							
Romanian Deadlift (1 leg)	set 1	6	6	8	8	10	10
	set 2	6	6	8	8	10	10
PB Reverse Crunch	set 1	12	12	15	15	18	18
	set 2	12	12	15	15	18	18
SUPERSET							
Cable Chopping	set 1	8	8	6	6	4	4
	set 2	8	8	6	6	4	4
DB Curl-to-Press	set 1	6	6	5	5	4	4
	set 2	6	6	5	5	4	4

THE CORE WORKOUT (CONT.)

Phase 4: Mixed (Weeks 10, 11, and 12—Week 13 Reload!)
Goals: Speed, Power, Strength, Quality

MOVEMENT PREP

MOVEMENT PREP A	Week 1	Week 2	Week 3
Forward Lunge/Forearm-to-Instep	1 × 5@	1 × 6@	1 × 7@
Backward Lunge with a Twist	1 × 5@	1 × 6@	1 × 7@
Calf Stretch	1 × 10@	1 × 12@	1 × 7@
Hand Walk	1 × 5	1 × 6	1 × 7
Inverted Hamstring	1 × 5@	1 × 6@	1 × 14@

MOVEMENT PREP B	Week 1	Week 2	Week 3
Hip Crossover	1 × 10@ to 90° knees	1 × 12@ to longer legs	1 × 7@ to straight legs
Scorpion	1 × 10@	1 × 12@	1 × 7@
Lateral Lunge	1 × 5@	1 × 6@	1 × 7@
Drop Lunge	1 × 5@	1 × 6@	1 × 7@
Sumo Squat-to-Stand	1 × 5	1 × 6	1 × 7
Prehab Hip: Glute Bridge (1 leg)	1 × 10@	1 × 12@	1 × 14@

PREHAB

PREHAB: SHOULDER	Week 1	Week 2	Week 3
PB *Y*	1 × 10 + 1 weight	1 × 12 + 1 weight	1 × 12 + 1 weight
PB *T*	1 × 10 + 1 weight	1 × 12 + 1 weight	1 × 12 + 1 weight
PB *W*	1 × 10 + 1 weight	1 × 12 + 1 weight	1 × 12 + 1 weight
PB *L*	1 × 10 + 1 weight	1 × 12 + 1 weight	1 × 12 + 1 weight

PREHAB: CORE	Week 1	Week 2	Week 3
Pillar Bridge Front/Opp Arm/Leg	2–3 × 20 sec.	2–3 × 30 sec.	2–3 × 40 sec.
Pillar Bridge Side (right/left) w/Abduction	2–3 × 20 sec.	2–3 × 30 sec.	2–3 × 40 sec.
Pillar Bridge Side (right/left) w/Adduction	2–3 × 20 sec.	2–3 × 30 sec.	2–3 × 40 sec.

ELASTICITY

ELASTICITY A	Week 1	Week 2	Week 3
Reactive Stepup	2 × 5@	2 × 6@	2 × 6@
Side-to-Side Jump-to-Sprint	4 × 6 jumps each side	4 × 5 jumps each side	4 × 6 jumps each side

ELASTICITY B	Week 1	Week 2	Week 3
Lateral Bound	2 × 6@	2 × 7@	2 × 8@
3-Hurdle Drill	3 × 8 sec.	4 × 8 sec.	4 × 10 sec.

ESD

Workout	Total/# Reps	Warmup	Work/Zone	Rest/Zone
10 Lactate Mixed	11 min./10 reps	3 min./Z1	15 sec./Z3	30 sec./Z1
11 Lactate Mixed	15 min./4 reps	3 min./Z1	1½ min./Z3	1½ min./Z1
3 Aerobic/Recovery	—	—	30+ min./Z1	—

REGENERATION (Done Anytime/Anywhere!)

Exercise	Week 1	Week 2	Week 3
Foam Hamstring	1 × 8@	1 × 10@	1 × 12@
Foam IT Band	1 × 8@	1 × 10@	1 × 12@
Foam Quad/Groin	1 × 8@	1 × 10@	1 × 12@
Foam Glute	1 × 8	1 × 10	1 × 12
Foam Back/Lat	1 × 8@	1 × 10@	1 × 12@
AIS Rope Calf	1 × 8@	1 × 10@	1 × 12@
AIS Rope Hamstring	1 × 8@	1 × 10@	1 × 12@
AIS Rope or Static IT/Glute	1 × 8@	1 × 10@	1 × 12@
AIS Rope Adductors	1 × 8@	1 × 10@	1 × 12@
AIS Rope or Static Quad/Hip	1 × 8@	1 × 10@	1 × 12@
AIS Shoulder (Side-Lying)	1 × 8@	1 × 10@	1 × 12@
AIS Rope Triceps	1 × 8@	1 × 10@	1 × 12@
AIS 90/90 Stretch	1 × 8@	1 × 10@	1 × 12@
AIS Quadruped Rocking	1 × 8	1 × 10	1 × 12

If you're pressed for time, select the 4 AIS stretches that best target your problem areas.

ABOUT THE AUTHORS

MARK VERSTEGEN is recognized as one of the world's most innovative sports-performance experts. As the owner of Athletes' Performance—cutting-edge training centers in Tempe, Arizona, and Carson, California—he directs a 25-person team of performance specialists and nutritionists to train some of the biggest names in sports, including soccer star Mia Hamm; baseball's Nomar Garciaparra, Roberto Alomar, and Vernon Wells; WTA tennis players Meghann Shaughnessy and Mary Pierce; golfers Jim Carter and Billy Mayfair; NFL veteran Trace Armstrong; hockey goalie Nikolai Khabibulin; and NBA forward Rick Fox.

By teaching an integrated lifestyle and training program that blends strength, speed, flexibility, joint and "core" stability, explosion, elasticity, and mental toughness, Verstegen helps athletes become not only faster and stronger but also more powerful, flexible, and resistant to injury and long-term back, hip, and other joint problems.

Verstegen has helped dozens of football players improve their NFL draft stock through his training methods; the group includes first-rounders Kyle Turley, Leonard Davis, Levi Jones, Nick Barnett, Jordan Gross, and Kwame Harris.

Because of his cutting-edge techniques and up-to-date knowledge of sports performance, Verstegen is a sought-after consultant. He serves as director of performance for the NFL Players Association, is an advisor to Adidas, and serves as a consultant to numerous athletic governing bodies, including the U.S. Tennis Association.

A dynamic speaker, Verstegen travels the world to address groups such as the American College of Sports Medicine, the National Strength and Conditioning Association, and many corporate events.

Verstegen and his training methods have been profiled in dozens of publications, including *Sports Illustrated, USA Today, Smithsonian, The Sporting News, ESPN: The Magazine, USA Today Baseball Weekly, Street and Smith's SportsBusiness Journal, Robb Report, Outside, Men's Journal, Golf Digest,* and *Scientific American.*

Verstegen was a walk-on linebacker at Washington State University who turned to performance coaching after a career-ending neck injury. After earning a bachelor's degree in exercise science from WSU and a master's degree in sports science from the University of Idaho, he became the assistant director of player development at Georgia Tech. In 1994, he created the International Performance Institute on the campus of the IMG Sports Academy in Bradenton, Florida, and was quickly recognized as an innovator in sports performance. In 1999, he moved to Phoenix to build Athletes' Performance, a world-class, independent training facility. The 30,000-square-foot complex recently was honored as the "facility of merit" by *Athletic Business* magazine for its design.

Verstegen and his wife Amy, a former Washington State soccer player, live in Scottsdale, Arizona.

PETE WILLIAMS is a contributing writer to *Street & Smith's SportsBusiness Journal* and *USA Today Sports Weekly.* He has written about fitness and performance for numerous publications, including *Muscular Development* and *Mind and Muscle Power,* and is the author of two books on the sports-memorabilia business: *Card Sharks* and *Sports Memorabilia for Dummies.* A graduate of the University of Virginia, he lives in Florida with his wife, Suzy, and son, Luke.

FURTHER READING

Boyle, Michael, *Functional Training for Sports*, Champaign, Ill.: Human Kinetics, 2003.

Cook, Gray, *Athletic Body in Balance*, Champaign, Ill.: Human Kinetics, 2003.

Mattes, Aaron, *Active Isolated Stretching*, Sarasota, Fla.: Aaron Mattes Therapy, 1995 (available at www.stretchingusa.com).

Wharton, Jim, and Phil Wharton, *The Whartons' Stretch Book,* New York: Times Books, 1996.

PHOTO CREDITS

INDEX

Boldface references indicate photographs or illustrations. <u>Underscored</u> page references indicate boxed text.

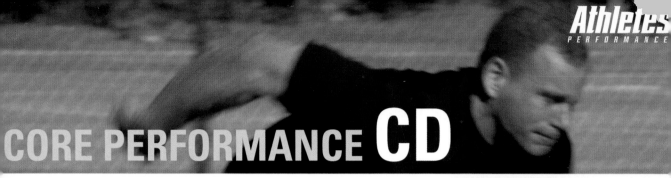

CORE PERFORMANCE CD

Athletes
PERFORMANCE

01	02	03
CORE WORKOUT	**CORE EXERCISES**	**CORE NUTRITION**
TRAINING METHODS	THE STEPS YOU TAKE	FUEL FOR PERFORMANCE

REVOLUTIONARY INTERACTIVE INSTRUCTION TO SUPPLEMENT YOUR CORE PERFORMANCE TRAINING

-> Over 150 video clips—featuring every exercise covered in the book

-> Printable versions of each workout and exercise

-> Printable journal sheets to track progress

-> Book section summaries

-> Sample recipes based on the Core Performance Nutrition Program

-> Much more!

! BY **ORDERING** THE **CORE PERFORMANCE CD** TODAY, YOU ARE AUTOMATICALLY ENTERED TO WIN A **FREE** WEEK OF **TRAINING AT ATHLETES' PERFORMANCE.**

Learn more about Athletes' Performance at www.athletesperformance.com